SENIORS ON THE MOVE

A GUIDE TO QUALITY OF LIFE AND LONGEVITY

For Sue

[signature] Jan. 20/24

ISBN: 978-0-9813616-9-7(PAPER BACK)
        978-0-9959933-0-3 (E-PUB)
        978-0-9959933-1-   (MOBI)

PUBLISHED BY AUTHOR

SENIORS ON THE MOVE

AUTHOR BIOGRAPHY

The author is 68 years old, semi-retired after 47 years in the retail grocery industry, and currently resides in Calgary, Alberta, Canada.

Inspired by the 1976 Olympic Games in Montreal, he was driven to take up the sport of distance running. He completed his first marathon in 1977, and it was the beginning of a career in endurance racing that would last over 35 years. Over that period, finish lines were crossed in over 30 marathons, two fifty-mile races, countless 10k races, and 11 Ironman triathlons.

Preparation for these endurance events included several decades of researching and implementing various training methods, diets, and optimum nutrition choices. Swimming, biking, running, and weight training were basically a way of life for decades. The knowledge of what training methods and food choices worked best was gained first-hand over years of intensive training and racing.

The author does not claim to be a professional athlete, coach, doctor, or nutritionist but rather, is sharing the knowledge gained from decades of training and racing.

Once his competitive career was over, the author created a website called www.Ironstruck.com that has been up and running for over 12 years.

He also self-published five books. Three books focus on inspiring, motivating, and providing training and racing tips for triathletes. He also wrote a lifestyle book for teens and pre-teens that features, adopting sound nutrition choices and regular exercise in everyday life. The fifth book was autobiographic in nature, about how embracing endurance sports changed the author's life for the better.

Although the author no longer competes, staying fit still remains the main focus. He still runs several times a week, does weight training on a regular basis, and maintains a healthy diet.

INTRODUCTION

As you settle into the retirement years, do you find yourself thinking more and more about the life you led?

Perhaps, you think about the glory days of your youth. Everything was so new, and there was so much to experience and learn. You had a thirst for life. You were invincible. Growing old was something your parents did, but not you. But in the blink of an eye, your life flashes by and suddenly, you're a senior.

In your journey through adulthood, you learned that life was full of choices. Do you often think about the decisions you made? Are you one of the lucky ones who has no regrets? If you had it all to do over again, are you certain you would never change a thing? Chances are you're like the majority of people, and wish you could go back and make at least, a few better choices.

Did you choose a career path that was far from what you really wanted to do with your life? Instead of taking a chance and reaching for the stars, you took the safer route. Perhaps, your true passion was just too risky and the challenge too great. You chose the smooth, paved highway, instead of the rocky road less travelled. Ultimately, you spent most of your working life doing a job you really didn't like. The longer you stayed at your job, the harder it was to give up the security, seniority, and all those holiday weeks you built up. Very often, you think wistfully at what might've been, if only you had been more courageous.

Did you build wealth and material trappings but ignore fitness and a healthy diet for most of your adult life? Are you unhappy with the reflection you see in the mirror?

Often, you think of the opportunity lost, and wish you had another chance to pursue your true calling, and take better care of yourself. We almost all have regrets that haunt us as we look back on our past. It's one of the mysterious realities of life; how ill-conceived decisions we make or singular moments of self-doubt can dictate the course of our lives. Yet, all is not lost.

Although, the errors of the past may be irrevocable, the opportunity to change for the better during the golden years of life is there for the taking. We can't alter yesterday, but we can certainly embrace today, and strive for a rewarding tomorrow full of accomplishments and realized dreams. It's never too late to find our better selves. What a worthy goal for all those who have no idea what to do with all their free time once they retire.

It's not too late to reach for the stars and do those things you convinced yourself were out of your reach. Learn that new language or that new skill. Go back to school. Learn how to dance. Give of yourself to others in need. Open that small business you always dreamed of having.

Most of all, commit yourself to a nutrition and fitness regimen that will keep you physically strong, and your mind sharp for years to come. Optimizing your physical and mental capabilities is the foundation that supports the dreams and goals you have for retirement.

Believe in yourself. You are capable of so much more than you might think. You'll simply be amazed at how quickly your body will respond to your efforts to embrace a healthier lifestyle.

As you enter into your senior years, you are not necessarily nearing the end of your existence. Dream big, and you might well be at the very beginning of the best years of your life. Regardless of the errors and missed opportunities of the past, you have the option to wake up any given morning and commit to living the rest of your life regret free.

CONTENTS

CHAPTER ONE

FITNESS FIRST

Did you ever wonder why many people find it so difficult to stay physically fit?

Did you ever wonder why people struggle so mightily with dieting and controlling their weight? I believe it's partly because North American society is built on a foundation of instant gratification. Why cook balanced meals when fast food is everywhere? Many crave the instant *high* that comes from booze, drugs, and random sex. Or perhaps, they want to be rich and reap the benefits of love and happiness without putting in the time and effort.

Throughout their lives, people are bombarded with the importance of exercising regularly. They see it everywhere. It actually begins in the earliest school years. All through their adult life, it's in newspapers, books, broadcast and social media. Yet, despite it all, there are many who just can't quite get a handle on it. It's such a struggle for them to commit to a lifestyle of health and fitness.

Often, taking care of one's health and wellbeing is relegated to the back burner.

Many people begin exercising with the best of intentions but they don't see results fast enough. They give up on including fitness into their lives because the gratification isn't instant. As a New Year's resolution, they buy fitness club memberships, swim passes, or exercise equipment, and try it for a while. They discover that it takes effort on their part. It takes them out of their comfort zone. All they have to show for a few excursions into the world of fitness is sore, and tired muscles, and disillusionment. As a result, they give up on exercising way too soon.

In years past, it may not have seemed such a big deal to let those New Year's resolutions slide after just a few weeks. Who cares if those fitness club memberships and swim passes expired virtually unused? So what if the basement or garage has become a graveyard for exercise equipment. Books and boxes are piled on your weight bench, and your exercise bike has become a clothes horse. At least you tried, didn't you?

However, if your age is taking you closer to senior territory, or if you're already a senior, there's not much wiggle room left for procrastination. If you want to get the most out of your senior years, it's important to understand that embracing a healthy lifestyle is the cornerstone of quality of life and longevity.

You can have all the money in the world set away for retirement. You can live in the biggest house on the highest hill. You can have brilliant plans for what should be the best years of your life. However, your overall health and fitness should come first or your exit could be an early one. Maybe you think it's too late for you. You're convinced there's not enough time for you to firm up your soft muscles, revitalize your cardiovascular system, strengthen your lungs, and regain the energy and stamina of years gone by.

The good news is that, it's never too late to start. It doesn't matter if you're 60 or 70 or 85. It's never too late to take that first step toward a new, improved you.

Keep in mind that it took you many years to get into your current physical condition. You won't necessarily see results after a few workouts. However, you'll be amazed how quickly your body will respond if sent signals that it's time to get moving. Stick with it, and change for the better will happen. Muscles that are sore at first will stop hurting, and instead, will get stronger. Your heart will strengthen as well to meet the demands of circulating blood to your working muscles.

Every time you walk, run, bike, swim, or lift a weight, your body responds to the challenge. Your heart, lungs, and muscles will pick up on the message that this is the way it's going to be. This is the new you. You will be sending the message that there's still much to do.

There was a time, not that long ago, when people who suffered heart attacks were told to sit back and take it easy, and not stress their weak hearts. There's an entirely new philosophy now. People who suffer heart attacks in this day and age are set in motion as soon as they are able. They begin to rack up the walking mileage and most eventually, begin to exercise on a regular basis. The goal after a heart attack now is to strengthen the heart as opposed to letting it remain in a weakened state. After all, the heart is a muscle, and will get stronger if challenged to perform.

If it happens that you're afflicted by disease, you can fight back or you can give in. It's pretty widely accepted now that regular fitness is the ultimate weapon against disease. It's not a matter of keeping up with others. It's a matter of challenging your body within your own set of circumstances and to the best of your ability.

Of course, there are no guarantees in this life. Even the fittest of us can be taken from this earth at any time. All we can do as seniors is give ourselves the best possible odds of living as many years as we can. The goal isn't to just survive, but rather, to live long and realize a quality of life that enables us to enjoy all the well-earned rewards of retirement.

Talk to your doctor about it. He'll most likely be thrilled that you want to make regular exercise a part of your life. Start today, and begin your journey toward positive change.

CHAPTER TWO

LIFE EXPECTANCY

Life expectancy is a statistical phenomenon. You could still be hit by the proverbial bus tomorrow-Ray Kurzweil

In 1980, the life expectancy for men and women in Canada was 70 and 74 respectively. You can add about ten years onto those figures by today's (2017) standards.

The United States is very much the same, but in recent years, their life expectancy took a bit of an unsettling dip. According to Scientific American, it appears that much of it has to do with more people dying which in turn, lowers the life expectancy rate.

In 2014 and 2015, drug overdoses and severe flu were being considered as two of the main causes of the increased death rate in the United States. It's sort of a grey area, because there was an increase in stroke and heart disease related death as well. If someone with heart issues contacted the flu, it could ultimately lead to their death.

Although there is no absolute evidence, it wouldn't be a stretch at all to consider obesity and lack of overall fitness as likely candidates when it comes to heart disease related deaths. It's no secret that obesity has pretty reached near epidemic proportions in North America. According to a 2016 article in the Toronto Sun, two-thirds of Canadians are either overweight or obese.

The news isn't all bad. Most insurance companies use a standard life expectancy chart similar to these stats posted by Sunlife Insurance. These are the results I came up with by using their parameters.

If a 65 year old 5'10" male weighs 250 lbs, smokes, has 3-5 drinks a day, has high blood pressure, and is physically inactive; life expectancy is 75 years. If this male has never smoked, it becomes 80 years.

If this same male has normal blood pressure, has 2 or less drinks a day, never smoked or quit smoking, and exercises several times per week; life expectancy is 88 years. Even if this person weighs 170 lbs, never smokes, and doesn't drink, their life expectancy tumbles to 83 years if they have high blood pressure, and are physically inactive.

For a 5'6" 150 lbs female who is 65 years old, has 3-5 drinks a day, high blood pressure, smoker, and physically inactive; life expectancy is 76 years. If all else is equal but her blood pressure is normal, she has 2 or less drinks a day, quit smoking or non-smoker, and exercise several times per week; life expectancy is a whopping 90 years.

Even if this person weighs 120lbs, never smokes, and doesn't drink, their life expectancy tumbles to 84 years if they have high blood pressure, and are physically inactive.

Regardless of statistics or where on earth you happen to live, there's one undeniable truth. Making the best possible nutrition choices, and adopting a lifestyle that includes physical fitness activity on a regular basis will give a person the best chance to live a long, healthy, and productive life.

It doesn't mean you have to be super skinny. As the stats show, a male who weighs 250 pounds, doesn't smoke, has normal blood pressure, and includes regular fitness in his life can add eight years to his life expectancy.

Sure, we've all heard the stories of some men who bombarded their bodies with smoking and drinking, and lived to be 100. Certainly, they are the exception rather than the rule, and may have been blessed with longevity enabling genes. At the same time, a man might do everything right and die at 80 years old. There are no guarantees in life. Ultimately, we should just give ourselves every possible advantage, and let the chips fall where they may.

Women seem to have the upper hand when it comes to longevity. According to Tom Perls, founder of the New England Centenarian Study at Boston University,

"across the industrialized world, women still live 5 to 10 years longer than men. Among people over 100 years old, 85% are women."

Some experts believe it's because men usually have to deal with heart attacks and strokes earlier than women. Instead of 50 or 60, women are more prone to deal with these problems when they're 70 or 80.

I think there's also another reason the longevity scale tips to the female side. Just think of all the times you hear about gang violence, bar room fights, overdoses, and car accidents caused by drunk drivers. More often than not, it involves men. Young males are often ruled by testosterone that makes them more prone to taking risks that could cost them their lives. Almost all soldiers who die in battle are males. Regardless of the reason, more deaths means a decline in the male longevity average.

Men are more stubborn as well when it comes to sickness. They will put off seeing a doctor almost until it's too late, whereas women are more apt to take better care of themselves. Women living longer than men is not just a North American phenomena. Women score highest on the longevity scale everywhere.

How about this for a statistic? The 2017 life expectancy for women living in Monaco is 93.45 years. The overall average for men and women combined is 89.42 years. Both statistics are number one in the world. So if you want to find out how to live long as possible, it appears that you have two choices. You can finish reading this book or move to Monaco.

CHAPTER THREE

RUN FOR YOUR LIFE

Every year, I come across more and more stories about retired seniors who take up running for the first time and then, become hooked on it. They start running for a number of reasons. Some run as a way to stay fit, and some run as a way to use up all that extra time on their hands. Something happens along the way. They're bitten by the running bug much like I was, way back in 1976.

Before they know it, they find themselves entering local 5K and 10K races. For some, that's not enough and one day, they find themselves at the start line of a marathon. Some senior runners end up expanding their horizons, and they run in races all over the country. They check online to see if there are any races happening in Hawaii or Great Britain when they plan on being there for a vacation.

Many dedicated senior runners are still running in their 80's, and in some cases, even their 90's. To me, it shows how embracing a lifestyle of regular fitness improves quality of life and longevity. So what is it about running that attracts people of all ages? Perhaps, people are drawn to the sense of well-being from endorphins released from being in motion. Maybe they realize the benefit of heart, lungs, and muscles, all working in harmony like a finely-tuned engine.

The surprising thing is that running wasn't even that popular 40 years ago. It was a male-dominated sport that seemed to attract a selected group of athletes. Running for women wasn't even on the distant horizon. Sure, there were some women running but not many. Then something remarkable happened in the mid 60's that made the world take notice of the female runner.

It was 1966 when a 23-year-old woman named Roberta "Bobbi" Gib, sent in an entry for the Boston Marathon. She was so excited when she got a letter back. However, her excitement was short-lived because this is what the letter said.

"This is an AAU Men's Division race only," wrote *race director Will Cloney. "Women aren't allowed, and furthermore are not physiologically able."*

Gib was pretty damn mad, and decided to go anyway. Not to be deterred, she hid in some bushes near the start line, and snuck into a large pack of runners when the gun went off. She was a sensation all along the course because no woman had ever run in the Boston Marathon. She crossed the finish line as an unofficial entrant in 3 hours, 21 minutes, and 40 seconds. A Sports Illustrated article perhaps said it best.

"Last week a tidy-looking and pretty 23-year-old blonde [had] a performance that should do much to phase out the old-fashioned notion that a female is too frail for distance running."

It opened the door for the female runner to be taken seriously and in 1984, the first women's Olympic Marathon took place in Los Angeles, and the rest as they say, is history. These days, there are pretty much as many female runners as there are male in any given race.

The running craze went ballistic in the 1980's, and has never stopped. It's not unusual today to see 10,000 entries in a big city marathon. Pretty much every city in the world has running races of varying distances. The birth of the internet was game-changing. People around the world had access to all things running. They could find information on equipment, training, coaching, racing, and diets.

I told this story for a reason. Millions of people can't be wrong. They took up running and ultimately, embraced the feeling of well-being, social interaction, and sense of accomplishment that are synonymous with the sport.

Running on a regular basis as seniors will do wonders for overall health. Staying mobile challenges the heart and lungs to work at optimum levels, and it improves the entire cardiovascular system. Of course, if running is new to you, it will take time to ease into it.

If you plan on getting into running for the first time or after a long layoff from the days when you used to run a lot, it's best to begin with a walk/run routine anyway. For example, walk for five minutes, and run easily for one minute. Repeat this a few times, depending on your level of ability. If you did three repeats, it would be an 18 minute cardiovascular workout that would include 15 minutes of walking, and three minutes of running.

As you get fitter, you can increase the degree of difficulty in several ways. You can decrease the time spent walking and run more, you can increase the number of repeats, or you can increase your speed. Months down the road, your walk/run workouts might become a 30 or 40 minute run. Half the fun is setting up your own program dependant on what your goals are. The important thing is to get started, and make physical fitness a regular part of your life.

There are several options when deciding where to run. You can run on a city bike path, on the side of the road or on an indoor or outdoor track. The important thing is to just get moving.

Of course, running isn't for everyone. Some people have weight issues, problems with their knees, or any number of reasons why running won't suit them.

Never fear.

Developing a regimen of walking on a regular basis with health and fitness in mind is an excellent option. Read on, and we'll have a look at the benefits of walking.

CHAPTER FOUR

WALK WITH PURPOSE

There are few physical traits more natural to human beings than walking and running. Most of us started walking when we were around 12 or 14 months old. Before long, those first few hesitant steps morphed into a run. Walking and running became our primary method of traveling from point A to point B.

Somewhere along the journey of life, walking substantial distances in everyday life may have fallen by the wayside. Perhaps, the typical day most of your adult life included walking to the car, subway, or bus and then, to your desk where you spent eight hours at a sedentary job.

Of course, that's not everyone.

There are those who walked a lot. They were on their feet all day at work or perhaps, went hiking on a regular basis. All in all, they led a healthy lifestyle.

Unfortunately, in this day and age, that's not most people. Obesity and lack of fitness has reached epidemic proportions in North America. The sad part is that it carries over into the senior years. It leaves people ill-prepared in the battle against a host of diseases that we are susceptible to as we age.

The good news is that it's never too late to take control of your wellbeing. Walking with purpose like running, is a great way to lose weight and improve your overall fitness. By walking with purpose, I mean that you incorporate a regular regimen of walking into your life.

You set up a program that includes walking specific distances as a means to an end. In other words, you're not just ambling out to the garage or over to the corner store. You're walking a set distance at a brisk pace with the specific purpose of working your heart, lungs, and muscles to the point that they become stronger and more efficient.

Everyone is at a different level when it comes to fitness. The key is to set up a walking plan that's doable for you. Once you've established how far you can walk in comfort, walk that distance over and over until you feel ready to increase it incrementally.

For example, if you walk 200 meters several times and it feels good, increase the distance a little. Over time, your 200 meters could well become half a mile or a mile. Eventually, you'll reach the ideal distance that suits you perfectly. In other words, that will be the average distance that you walk several times a week. At this point, you don't really have to increase the distance any more unless you choose to. There's a way to get more out of your weekly walks without increasing the distance you travel.

Our caveman ancestors ran and walked in short bursts during the hunt and then, rested and ran again. Basically, it was much like we call interval training these days. Instead of walking great distances at a slow pace, it would be more beneficial to incorporate intervals of faster walking followed by your regular slower pace.

Raising and lowering your heart rate as you alternate between fast and slow is ideal for strengthening your heart. People sometimes forget that the heart is a muscle that needs to be challenged in order to stay strong.

On the off days from your longer, walks you might walk a shorter distance, have a rest day, or do something else you enjoy in the way of fitness.

If you're starting a walking program for the first time, a good choice is to walk around your own block to begin with. This always keeps you close to home. As you become fitter and stronger, you can increase the number of trips around the block, or you can begin to walk further from home to add a little variety to the scenery.

Quite often, seniors will get together and hit one of the big malls early in the morning when they first open. They'll walk a pre-determined amount of laps around all the shops and then, go for breakfast. Not a bad way at all to spend a morning.

I think this is an especially great idea on those cold winter days. There's no reason you can't walk with others as long as you and your companions are comfortable with the pace. It's no fun to be walking a pace that you struggle with.

Pay special attention to your footwear. Invest money in a good pair of walking shoes that feel really comfortable. I would suggest going to a shoe store and have someone knowledgeable find the ideal length and width for you. The last thing you need is to walk substantial distances in shoes that don't fit you properly.

Choose your clothing carefully as well. Be sure to wear clothes that have fairly loose fitting, and appropriate for the ever-changing temperature and weather conditions.

 If you're planning on walking for quite a long way, be sure to take along a cell phone, something to snack on, and water. For example, I've run into seniors who walk for miles and are gone for most of the day. Some people really love it, and will walk to different parts of the city and see things that sort of whiz by unnoticed when you're in a car. They'll stop for coffee, breakfast, or lunch and walk some more.

Some seniors who have become very fit even take to hiking through the mountains, or walking trails in far off countries.

It was easy to put regular exercise on the back-burner when you were thirty or forty something. There just wasn't enough time in your busy schedule, and there was always next year anyway, wasn't there?

If you're retired, you probably have tons of time on your hands. What a perfect time to put on those walking shoes.

Regardless of your age, it's never too late to get started on the road to improved fitness. It's never too late to reap the rewards of immeasurable health benefits as you move forward, ever forward. The main thing is to take those first few steps toward a better way of life.

Once you experience the physical, mental, and emotional benefits that come part and parcel with regular exercise, you might never want to stop. You'll want to always continue the journey toward a new, improved you.

CHAPTER FIVE

TREADMILL TIPS

There are many advantages to having a good treadmill in your home. Although they can be quite expensive, it could well be one of the best investments you ever make. New treadmills can range in price anywhere from about $700 to $10,000. Often, there are used ones available for around $500.

Before purchasing a new or used treadmill, several things have to be taken into consideration. How much will the treadmill be used? How many people will be using it as this determines wear and tear? Will an entry level treadmill be good enough for your purposes?

There are people who get treadmills to aid in their marathon training, and might eventually put thousands of kilometers on their treadmill. Then there are seniors just wanting to begin walking or perhaps, running for fitness. This means the wear and tear on the treadmill will be less.

The amount of use and the weight of users often dictates the price and make of the treadmill. For instance, a heavier person might require a treadmill with a bigger motor. Someone training for a marathon would most likely want a wider running surface.

The treadmills you see at fitness centers are industrial models built to take constant abuse day after day. These are the high end models that can run into the thousands of dollars. Usually, they'll have a larger motor, and wider running surface. People of all sizes with different goals use fitness center treadmills, and it's sort of one size fits all. Serious runners, senior walkers, and those weighing 300-400 pounds or more might use that same treadmill.

It's not really necessary to spend thousands of dollars on these high end models. From all the research I've done, it appears that $1000 is about the ideal starting point for a good quality new treadmill for the home.

Something else to consider is that there are probably used treadmills for sale all over your city. Just check out Kijiji. You can save a lot of money because many people buy treadmills with the best of intentions and then, hardly use them. They weigh a lot and take up space, and people will sometimes, sell them at a good price just to have someone come pick them up, and get them out of their house.

The typical treadmill ad will usually read something like this....

Used treadmill for sale $500. Hardly used and like new. You must pick up and you'll need a pick-up truck and someone to help you because it's heavy.

Keep in mind that you'll need a couple of strong people with a large vehicle if you're picking up a used treadmill. By the same token, most stores will charge for delivery if you're buying new. There's also the matter of warranty. Most likely, you won't have one if you buy a used treadmill.

Whether you buy new or used, my suggestion would be to do your homework on treadmills if you're thinking it might be an option for you. You can do a search online, or visit a local store that specializes in fitness equipment. Most likely, they will have treadmills in a full range of prices, including high end industrial models. Of course, you don't have to buy a treadmill from them, but you can certainly ask questions.

The salesperson will probably ask the purpose of the treadmill to determine what size of motor or width of belt would be best for your exercise goals. Plus, you can have a look at several models and get some idea what features are included.

Getting as much information as you can will also come in handy if you decide to buy used. Most treadmill for sale ads will include the brand name and perhaps, the size of the motor and other features. It's to your advantage to learn as much as you can before purchasing a used model.

Another important consideration is just how much space it'll take up, and where to set it in your home. If you have a condo or apartment, it limits your choices. Most people set them up in their living room with sight lines to the T.V. That way, they can get lots of natural light and entertainment while they exercise. If you own a detached home, there are far more options. You can put a treadmill in the basement, in a spare bedroom, or even in a heated garage.

It might appear at first glance, that spending any length of time on a treadmill might be boring, but not necessarily so in this day and age, when you can listen to music on an I-pod or cell phone or tape your favorite T.V shows to entertain you as you train. Besides, you don't have to be on your treadmill for hours. If you're just doing a brisk walk or easy run for 25-30 minutes, you really don't have time to get bored.

If you're willing to dedicate yourself to a fitness program of walking or running, there are several advantages to treadmills. Many seniors might feel self-conscious if the whole concept of fitness is new to them. They might be frail, overweight, or just seriously out of shape. It would be far easier for them to exercise in the comfort of their own home.

There are also no limitations on when or how much you can use a treadmill. You can exercise year round, no matter what the weather's like outside. You can get on that treadmill and walk a few miles before breakfast, or fit in a workout late at night if you can't sleep. Best of all, you can also exercise at your own pace without feeling out of place or embarrassed.

A treadmill is versatile, and when your fitness improves, it's there for you if you want to graduate from walking to running. Many people combine walking and running outdoors along with indoor treadmill training. They might choose to do most of their walking or running outside, but when weather or time constraints are an issue, a treadmill is an ideal alternative.

Personally, I feel every retirement home should come complete with an exercise room that has free weights, weight training stations, exercise bikes, and treadmills.

When it comes to treadmills, I found this comment interesting as it indicates that fitness for seniors is considered important all over the world.

Research shows the fountain of youth may flow between the treadmill and dumbbells. "Muscles weaken with age; physical activity helps rejuvenate their stem cells and promote circulation," says Dafna Benayahu, a medical researcher at Tel Aviv University. "Regular workouts may undo signs of aging elsewhere in the body."

CHAPTER SIX

RESISTANCE TRAINING

"Don't use all your muscles, only the ones you want to keep."

It wasn't all that long ago when the weight lifting rooms of the world were dominated by testosterone-laden power lifters. They were huge guys with rippling muscles. Many people new to the world of squats, bicep curls, and leg extensions found it intimidating just to walk into a weight room. All they probably wanted was to try and improve themselves, but they felt conspicuous and out of place. I imagine it was even worse for seniors. That's probably why it was an oddity, just a couple of decades ago, to see someone with grey hair pumping iron with the rest of them.

Times have certainly changed. More and more seniors have discovered the benefits of lifting weights. There was an experiment done with a group of seniors living in a nursing home. Their ages were between 87 and 96. Remarkably, in just eight weeks of lifting weights, they increased their strength by almost 200%.

A University of Vermont study of healthy seniors, ages 65 to 79, found out that subjects could walk almost 40 percent farther without a rest after 12 weeks of weight training.

These seniors are perfect examples that it's very possible to regain muscles that were lost years before. There's a medical term for losing muscle mass as we age. It's called Sarcopenia. From about the mid-thirties, people slowly begin to lose muscle. The less active a person is, the more muscle they lose. The process begins to speed up around 65-75 years of age.

The best way to slow down this muscle loss is to make a concerted effort to get fitter and stronger. It can have a dramatic effect on a senior's quality of life.

Strengthening leg muscles is a powerful weapon against future disabilities, including the inability to walk. Just for that fact alone, I think all seniors should be involved in a strength training program.

Improving mobility is just the beginning of the benefits. By becoming stronger, balance and agility will improve. This can help prevent falls that seniors are often prone to. A study at Tufts University found that older women who lifted weights for a year improved their balance by 14 percent. (A control group composed of women who didn't lift weights suffered a 9 percent decline in balance in the same year.)

When you adopt a program of strength training, you're getting more than bigger, stronger muscles. The tendons and ligaments around all your joints are strengthened as well. Your range of motion is improved, and the pain people often feel in their joints is minimized. Everyday, challenges like walking and climbing stairs becomes easier.

Weight training and exercising in general can also have a positive effect on the brain. Neurotransmitters are stimulated during exercise. This reaction helps reduce or eliminate depression and other emotional stress that people encounter in the course of their everyday lives.

I know this for a fact from past experience. Often, after an invigorating workout, I felt this amazing high that no drug can provide. It was more like a sense of well-being. It was almost as if my body was saying, "thanks for looking after me".

If your body senses that muscles are not being used, it will basically let them fall into a state of disrepair. In other words, atrophy sets in. To put it bluntly, if you do nothing in the way of exercise or strength training as you age, your whole body essentially gets progressively weaker. That in turn opens you up to all sorts of medical issues. Your heart isn't the powerful muscle it once was, arteries harden, bones get brittle, and ability to function and do everyday tasks becomes increasingly difficult.

The good news is that your body is receptive to your efforts to become fitter. It senses activity, and the need to strengthen and improve. Your body becomes stronger to meet the new demands you're asking of it.

In one of my books, I called the human body a miracle of creation. Most people just take their bodies for granted, and don't understand how it reacts to every single thing they do. There's an example I like to use that pretty much defines what I'm trying to say.

If a person suddenly becomes blind, it's not long before the body compensates by fine tuning all the other senses. Although, most people have the ability to hear, taste, touch, and smell, they don't necessarily use them at full capacity. A blind person fine tunes those same senses to compensate for their lack of sight. The body adapts the remaining senses as a protection mechanism.

A better term for weight lifting or strength training is resistance training. You're pushing your body to do just a little more all the time. When you lift a weight, you want the muscles involved to reach a point where you meet resistance. Your body senses that the particular muscle being worked has to get stronger because you're asking it to do more than it's able to do efficiently. You're telling your body you need more strength.

The basic concept is really very simple when you first enter the world of resistance training involving weights. Whatever your age, sex, or current physical condition, it's important to begin an exercise with an amount of weight you can easily lift. Say for instance, you're doing bicep curls. Keep adding small amounts at a time until you reach the point where you can feel the resistance.

If you begin with one pound, and can do your bicep curl ten times with little effort, you should begin adding increasingly larger amount of weight until you feel that point of resistance. You'll know it because you have to work a little harder to do the exercise. The last two or three repetitions of a set of ten should take some work to complete. That's perfect.

Do the same exercise with the same amount of weight three days a week. Every other day is best because muscles require a rest day to rebuild. For example, you might train on Monday, Wednesday, and Friday with the weekend off.

Whatever weight lifting exercise you do, if you stick with it, you'll reach the point where you find it far easier to finish your ten repetitions. If you are able, I would suggest adding another set of ten to each workout once you've mastered the first set.

You may not be able to finish all ten of the second set. Just do what you can. If you dedicate yourself to your training on a regular basis, you'll eventually reach the point where you can finish both sets comfortably. That means you've become stronger.

Congratulations!

Now, put on a little more weight, and repeat the process. Look at it this way. If you started with one pound, and eight weeks later, you can do your two sets of ten repetitions with three pounds, you've pretty much tripled the strength of that particular muscle.

The same principle of adding weight incrementally is the very same if you are using resistance machines in a fitness facility. For example, I believe two of the more important exercises when it comes to strengthening leg muscles are leg extensions and hamstring curls. They work the big quad muscles in the front, and the hamstrings at the back of the leg.

By strengthening these muscles, you give added support to your knees. This does wonders for mobility. Seniors have been known to shock family and friends with how mobile they've become, and how far they can walk after six or eight weeks of improving leg muscle strength.

There's more than one method of resistance training.

There's also resistance training without weights. It's better known as Isometrics. If you push against a wall with both hands until you feel the resistance against your arms and shoulders, that's an example of isometrics. A push-up is an isometric exercise.

Prisoners locked up in cells often use the isometric method of training. Their weight machines are the steel bars, walls, and floor of their cell.

Fitness expert, Andre Read, has an excellent explanation of the difference between doing a specific exercise with a weight or through Isometrics.

"Muscle can only contract in a few ways. It can do the obvious and contract to shorten the distance between joints, such as when doing a bicep curl. This is called a concentric contraction, where the muscle tenses while shortening. It can also tense while lowering a load, or resisting it, such as when lowering the weight in a curl. This type of contraction is known as eccentric and occurs when the muscle tenses while lengthening. A final type of contraction is called an isometric contraction, and it occurs when the muscle tenses while not changing length. Examples of this are pushing against an immoveable object such as a wall."

Regardless if you're 60 or 90, resistance training can be instrumental in improving your quality of life. The trick is to let your body know that you're not ready to slow down or stop. Basically, you're the master telling your body what you want it to do.

CHAPTER SEVEN

SWIMMING WITH GRACE

By guest expert, Terry Laughlin, creator of the Total Immersion swim technique

Want to age gracefully? Swim gracefully—and mindfully.

How many individuals do you know who—nearing 70 years of age—are striving to achieve personal bests in a sport measured by time and distance? And how many people--in any age group--do you know who are pursuing improvement by regularly and rigorously analyzing what they do, seeking weaknesses, and trying to convert them into strengths?

Such behaviors are quite rare in the world at large—even among those in their 20s or 30s, let alone four decades older. However, they are surprisingly common, at all ages, in the community of Total Immersion swimmers.

The day I began writing this chapter, I received an email from Wayne Britton, 68, of Pembrokeshire, England. Wayne described himself as a 'recreational' swimmer, but his message made it evident that a more accurate description was *Kaizen* swimmer--one devoted to thoughtful self-examined, pursuit of continuous improvement.

Wayne learned front crawl from a traditional (non-TI) coach shortly before turning 60. Five years later, seeking more refined technique, he attended a Total Immersion Effortless Endurance workshop. At the conclusion of the workshop, Coach Tracey Baumann counted his strokes, and timed him for 25 meters. This gave Wayne a set of 'baseline' metrics—25 meters in 32 strokes and 46 seconds—data from which he could track improvement.

Over the next year, Wayne improved to 42 seconds and 26 strokes. Seeking to boost his progress, Wayne attended a TI Smart Speed workshop. While there, coaches Keith Lewis and Mike Weedon persuaded him to focus on developing a more streamlined stroke—and to let gains in speed be products of that, rather than being overt goals. Since then, he's improved his 25m stroke count to an average of 20 SPL (strokes per length) while swimming 50m repeats in 78 seconds.

At the present, Wayne's focus is on feeling more consistency in "moving through the water with a relaxed, graceful, no-splash stroke." Wayne has also begun working with a Tempo Trainer, which allows him to increase tempo in precise increments of .01 (one-hundredth) second at a time.

In this chapter, I'll make the case that swimming has truly unique properties and potentials that promote aging-with-grace. Let's begin with what is the common knowledge about swimming-and-aging: Few other physical activities are as ideally suited to accommodate the changes and challenges that come with age. Swimming is low-impact. It's aerobic. It works all our muscles in equal proportion. It keeps us both supple and well-toned.

You can gain those physical benefits simply by swimming regularly—say two to three times a week, for 30 minutes or more. However, by including some of the Kaizen habits of Wayne's swimming, you create the possibility of quite rare and valuable benefits, to brain and psyche. By pursuing improvement—rather than simply putting in hours or miles—you develop mindsets, habits, and behaviors that can keep you strong and supple in body *and* mind, and cultivate a positive, constructive attitude toward the aging process.

Improvement-Minded Swimming

To be a Kaizen swimmer, make it your primary goal to *improve your swimming* (not to 'get in the yards' or get your heart rate up) in every practice i.e. make and carry out a plan to *be a better swimmer* when you leave the pool than you were when getting in. Rather than have just added another mile to your total.

Swimming is uniquely suited for this approach because it offers almost limitless improvement possibility, even for those who start late in life. Dr. Paul Lurie took his first swim lesson, with me, at age 94. He was still improving his speed at age 97. At 99, he still strives to stroke as efficiently as possible in his daily 20-length (in a 50-foot pool) practice.

Our great improvement upside is due to the fact that--as an *aquatic* skill—swimming is an 'alien activity' for humans, after millions of years adapting to life on land. A measure of this was provided by a study, conducted in 2004 and published in 2005, by DARPA engineers.

Tasked with designing a swim foil for the Navy Seals, they studied the efficiency of dolphins and human swimmers. They found that dolphins convert 80% of energy into forward motion. Their human subjects—lap swimmers who'd received no coaching—averaged only 3% energy efficiency. Ninety-seven percent of their efforts were diverted into moving around in water, and moving the water around--rather than moving *through* water.

In teaching thousands of late-starting adults over the last three decades, we made an important discovery: Every solution to the most common sources of energy waste is utterly counter-intuitive. Every efficiency-promoting technique overturns a long-held idea--in many cases, even a primal instinct--about how to swim. This means that:

1. At the outset of your improvement process, you must reconcile a significant conflict in your 'mental model' for how to swim; and
2. On every stroke you take, you must be mindful in order not to be drawn back to inefficient instinct or habit. Swimming should be practiced as a form of moving meditation.

Both activities, it turns out, have been shown to promote a more 'youthful' brain.

What Can You Improve?

Your Mental Model

Each of us has a mental model—a framework of ideas and impressions--for how swimming 'works.' We assemble that model, over the course of a lifetime of experiences and exposures—is what we hear from others and what we see them do. Much of the framework gradually becomes sub-conscious, unexamined, and reflexive. For example:

- We go to the pool and—out of habit or a lack of other ideas--reflexively swim a continuous mile.

- We push off the wall on each lap, focused mainly on *getting to the other end*—not so much on how we get there.
- If we're among the relatively small number who think about technique, we're likely to focus on how we pull and kick.
- When we get tired, we conclude it's from a lack of conditioning, and we resolve to swim longer and/or harder.

Then we encounter something—perhaps, this chapter—that causes us to re-examine long-held ideas. We are made more curious, and realize much about swimming, that it isn't as it has always seemed.

As a result, our mental model evolves, and we go to the pool with a conscious goal of working on skills, cultivating greater sensory awareness, and strengthening our capacity for focus. What was formerly a workout, is now a *practice*.

- We push off the wall with a *mental blueprint* for the technique that will most efficiently carry us to the other end. On every stroke, we compare blueprint to what we're feeling, and assess by how much we've missed the mark. At the next wall, we adjust our thinking process, attempting to align reality with blueprint.

- Our technique focus is on shaping the body to minimize drag, rather than maximize propulsion.
- We counter fatigue by striving to reduce energy waste, rather than continuously topping up a seriously leaky tank of muscle fuel. We redefine endurance to "the ability to repeat fluent, relaxed swimming movements for as long as we like".

Your Technique

Guided by the Total Immersion 'Pyramid' of technique foundations, you establish a clear set of priorities in developing your technique. This pyramid provides clarity on the order in which to acquire skills—start with the base and work your way up—and on the relative importance of each step: The more volume in each step, the more practice time and attention you should devote to it.

The steps in the pyramid are:

Balance

Balance is the foundation upon which you build a *robustly* efficient stroke—one that not only minimizes energy waste, but also resists breakdown as you add distance or speed. When you master the skill of Balance, you achieve a kind of *nirvana* of feeling completely comfortable under water, and having real control over your body position. You'll understand what causes that sinking sensation, and how to shift to a feeling of weightlessness—via a clever application of physics principles, instead of kicks and heartbeats.

Balance skills provide immediate and dramatic energy savings. They are the simplest of all swimming skills to learn because they involve the largest body parts and muscle groups—easy to coordinate and easy to sense. Finally, they enable mastery of all subsequent skills. Without Balance, everything you do will be compromised. With it, you'll find it almost ridiculously easy to master the skills that follow.

Streamlining

Once you've balanced your body, then shape it to be more *fishlike*. Eons of evolution have given fish and aquatic mammals the ideal shape for moving through water—a sleek 'uni-body,' tapered at either end, with a minimum of moving parts. In contrast, humans have evolved for stability and mobility on land, with parts that—when we swim according to instinct (head high to avoid choking and all four limbs churning to avoid sinking)-- create a 'perfect storm' of drag and turbulence.

Fortunately, the human brain—with its awesome problem-solving capabilities--is up to the task of what we call 'vessel shaping' to reshape the body to

(i)   Arrive in its most hydrodynamic position as we complete each stroke; and
(ii) Maintain that highly streamlined position for more of each stroke cycle.

However, without the evolved mental map that prioritizes streamlining, and the patience to learn the necessary skills, we'll continue to churn up a storm of drag.

After Balance skills, Streamlining skills are next in order of payback. They provide massive energy savings with almost no energy cost to perform. And, because reshaping the body relies mostly on the largest body parts and muscle groups, they can be learned relatively quickly.

Propulsion (Move as One)

We teach propulsion skills last because:

1. They require more coordination and self-awareness to master.
2. They impose an energy cost.
3. They provide far less payback in efficiency or speed gains.

When teaching introductory Propulsion skills, we focus mainly on getting the head, arms, and legs to move in synchronization. Synchronous body movement automatically improves propulsive efficiency—moving your *body* <u>forward</u>, rather than moving the water back. But, even more, it contributes to energy efficiency in two ways:

1. Increasing the overall grace and fluency of your movements—getting body parts to work together, rather than independently, and working *with*, not against, the water.
2. Developing a *core-body-driven* stroke, rather than an arms-driven stroke. The core is both far more powerful, and far more fatigue resistant. The arms are relatively weak and quite prone to fatigue.

Your Self-Awareness

Elite athletes appear different from the rest of us; they seem to have been born with distinct genetic advantages. The world's best freestyle swimmers are much taller than average, with supple joints, broad shoulders, and narrow hips. But elites also share a less obvious advantage over average athletes; they possess far greater sensory awareness. Swimming coaches call this "feel for the water" and speak of it as a little-understood— almost mystical—quality; a lucky few seem to have been born with it. The less fortunate just lacks it, and can do little more to change that than eye color or foot size.

However, in teaching late-starting adults for over 25 years, we've seen countless times that 'feel for the water' is *learnable*. You cultivate it by doing something that is almost never seen in traditional training programs—making Self-Sensing exercises a systematic and foundational element, given equal or greater importance with aspects like distance, time, and effort.

It's most immediate benefit is that—unlike physical characteristics such as size, body type, or fitness—average swimmers can equal or surpass elites in feel for the water by consciously trying to develop it. A holistic benefit is that it produces many of the salutary effects of mindfulness training (which is based on self-sensing of the breath, posture, mind-focus, etc.) and transforms tedious and repetitive training into an engaging and enjoyable activity.

3 Steps to Greater Awareness

Introduce Self-Sensing elements and tasks to your training via a 3-step process:

1. **Pay attention.** Create an *organized and prioritized* way to scrutinize specific aspects of your stroke. Choose a specific focal point—e.g. head-spine alignment—then focus on it intensely and tirelessly. At first, you'll discover this is quite challenging. But, like maintaining focus in meditation, your ability to concentrate improves with practice. You'll also find that it makes any lap, practice—or race--more enjoyable.

2. **Notice and compare.** When 'targeted' attention becomes a habit, you'll begin to notice

subtle, previously-overlooked, sensations. This feedback can be invaluable to improving elements of stroke efficiency like drag-reduction and stroke-synchronization. Once you create formal feedback loops, begin to assess what this feedback means, and how to respond: Do you swim faster with more ease, or fewer strokes? Does one focus make your stroke feel better overall than another? Wayne employs both forms of feedback.

3. **Make informed choices.** Use this new information to make more effective choices. This transforms formerly generic or "one-size-fits-all" training into a personalized problem-solving exercise. This adds a sense of purpose to the engagement and enjoyment produced by the mindfulness part of Self-Sensing training.

Your Ability to Coach Yourself

A natural outcome of pursuing these improvement projects--in Mental Model, Technique, and Awareness—is that you develop a sense of autonomy or empowerment. You feel less dependent on outside experts to guide your development as a swimmer. You feel a new confidence in setting meaningful goals, and knowing how to achieve them. Pursuing incremental, steady improvement becomes second nature—and a source of passion for swimming.

I'm not suggesting that you no longer seek coaching. Roger Federer, whose tennis strokes are the most beautiful in the world, has a stroke coach. Shouldn't you? And the first principle of Mastery is "Seek a Sensei". Rather, when you do engage with a coach, it's a partnership in which you accept equal responsibility for the quality of your learning experience and know how to maximize the value of time with the coach.

Even when you seek out specialized coaching— even as you stroke up and down the pool with a coach giving instruction and feedback—you'll be coaching yourself for the 20 or more seconds between instruction at the start of the length, and feedback at its end. And you'll resume coaching yourself entirely when you return to regular practice after meeting with a coach. So, expertise in Self-Coaching is an invaluable attribute. And an enormously satisfying one.

* * *

The Evolution of my 'Life Practice of Swimming'

I'm 66 years old; I've been swimming for over 50 years, and coaching for 45 years. If we peak physically in our late 20s, I've experienced nearly 40 years of aging effects on physical capacity. I viewed aging with trepidation when I was younger, but the older I've gotten, the more positively I view it. Especially as I've become eligible for 'senior' privileges and discounts, and moved from private medical insurance to Medicare in the last few years.

The high-water mark of my own swimming began at around age 50. Throughout my 40s, I taught myself TI techniques, often using myself as 'guinea fish' for the drills and techniques we taught in workshops.

I began competing again in Masters swimming, coming surprisingly close to my college times in my early 40s. However, my 'workouts' were still volume-and-effort oriented like in college.

After turning 50, I began to rely more on intuition. I only did practices I felt eager to do. I spent more time planning practices that maximize what I learn about my swimming, experimenting with many combinations of stroke count and tempo. I pushed myself to adapt to a much brisker tempos as Wayne is planning to do now, while maintaining an overall feeling of grace and flow, and an efficient stroke count. I also began to apply behavioral lessons and principles of Mastery and Deliberate Practice to everything about my swimming. I completed many marathon swims during my 50s, including the 28.5 mile Manhattan Island Marathon Swim in 2002 and 2006.

During these years, my passion and pleasure reached a strikingly higher level. As did my performance. Between 55 and 60, I became a Masters National Champion for the first time, eventually winning six national titles and breaking two national records in the 55-59 age group for the 1-Mile and 2-Mile Cable Swims in open water.

After turning 60, I continued to race regularly, striving instead to transform races into a 'work of art' rather than a competition with others. I completed several additional marathons, including a swim across Gibraltar Strait in Oct 2013, and from Corsica to Sardinia in Oct 2015.

My Illness-Free Zone

In Nov 2015, less than a month after completing a very strong, utterly tireless 10-mile swim from Corsica to Sardinia in 4 hours and 30 minutes, I was diagnosed with stage IV prostate cancer. In 18 months since—due to both advancing cancer and its treatment—I've experienced what seems like another 20 years of aging, in terms of loss of physical capacity, concentrated into less than two years.

During this period, I've continued racing, setting new 'lifetime slowest' marks in every race. But I've still taken great satisfaction in these races from aspects like maintaining an efficient stroke count, pacing expertly, and maintaining unblinking focus during pool events that last more than 26 minutes.

In the last two months, I've faced a new challenge. Each practice, as I begin swimming, I feel breathless and my chest burns, no matter how easily I swim. I seem to record slower times each week for short repeats like 100 yards. What do I do when that happens? I pay close attention to subtle sensations, analyze what I'm doing, look for weak points I can slightly strengthen.

By focusing on relaxing even more, on getting as much as possible out of each (gentle) stroke, within a few repeats, I can match the initial time with less discomfort . . . then coax out a tiny bit more speed . . . then maintain that faster pace for a longer distance. I could gradually stretch my initial 'breathless' 100-yard pace to 200, then 300, then 400--and once even 500--reasonably comfortable yards. No matter how many times I repeat this process—and no matter that the paces are slowing steadily--it feels as satisfying an accomplishment as anything I've done in 50 years of swimming.

In that way, I maintain an undiminished passion for swimming, my appetite for kaizen—between my initial repeat on a given evening and what follows—and find I can create what I call an 'illness-free' zone in the pool, in which I feel markedly healthier than at other times during the day.

My swimming, teaching, and work as a swimming educator and advocate—as in writing this guest chapter—help me sustain a 'lust for life' and a sense of mastery that invest every day with meaning and purpose. I'm certain that this is medicine equally strong to anything the doctors are giving me.

I'm most fortunate to have spent 25 years developing Kaizen habits and mindsets. At the time of my greatest need, they ensure that swimming remains a powerfully life-sustaining activity.

How to Start on a Kaizen Path

Total Immersion offers two downloadable Self-Coaching Courses for freestyle.

The <u>1.0 Effortless Endurance Freestyle Course</u> teaches the Pyramid skills of Balance,

Streamlining and Propulsion—which Wayne continues to refine.

The <u>2.0 Freestyle Mastery Course</u> teaches the advanced propulsion skills—plus Mastery in combining Stroke Length and Tempo--which Wayne is also working on.

Wayne is using both courses to guide his development and keep his improvement on track.

For a 10% saving, type **ironstruck** (no caps) in the coupon box on the Total Immersion website.

CHAPTER EIGHT

SICKNESS AND FITNESS

About twenty years ago, my father had a heart attack. Back then, he was told to take it easy and not do anything to stress his already weak heart. Two years later, he had another heart attack and died.

The approach to recovering from a heart attack or heart surgery is far different now. I often wonder how much longer my dad would've lived had he been encouraged to exercise and strengthen his heart instead of taking it easy.

These days, as soon as patients are able, they usually begin cardiac rehabilitation. I used to see them all the time, walking laps around the track at a local fitness center. They were being closely monitored by health care staff. I was impressed at the pace some of them were walking. To use one of my favorite terms, they were walking with purpose.

They seemed to be alternating between slower and faster laps which makes perfect sense. This is pretty much the same concept I mentioned in the previous chapter on walking. Making your heart work, and then resting it eventually, results in a stronger heart.

It's important that patients who are recovering from heart surgery find out from their doctor how to connect with rehab specialists if nobody has been in touch with them. Chances are their heart surgeon has already set them up with access to cardiac rehab sessions. Whatever the case, it's important to begin exercising under supervision once recovered from surgery.

The exercise of choice after surgery seems to be walking. It cost nothing, and it's very easy to monitor progress. Everybody is different and will have their own specific goals. To start with, patients are encouraged to do what they can manage. They might only be able to walk for a couple of minutes in the beginning. They start breathing hard and have to stop.

Over time, they get fitter and they increase the distance, and could well be exercising for 20 minutes after six or eight weeks. As they get stronger, they might choose to include different exercises. Swimming, biking, and resistance training are just a few options once their doctor gives the go ahead.

There are people who have exercised very little over the course of their lives. They're introduced to exercising as part of their rehab, and many begin to like the way it makes them feel. Some people actually become so fit that they get hooked on the feeling. Over the years, I've come across people who have recovered from a heart attack, and are entering marathons and triathlons. One marathoner said he'd never done any running at all until after he had a heart attack and was introduced to fitness out of necessity.

Certainly, it's depressing to have to deal with health issues, but they are a fact of life. There's little doubt that exercising is the key weapon against sickness. Being fit can be a difference maker when it comes to combating illness.

Heart issues, Cancer, Diabetes, Asthma, Celiac Disease, back problems, and painful joints would be a lot easier to deal with if fitness on a regular basis were part of the equation. It's also been well-documented that stroke victims can reduce vascular risk, and improve mobility. Regular exercise also improves balance, prevents muscle atrophy, improves blood flow, and most of all, does wonders for self-esteem.

I know first-hand how easy it would be to just throw in the towel when things aren't so great health wise. It was the year 2001 when I was at the top of my game as an endurance athlete. My goal was to be one of the best in my age-group in the Ironman Triathlon. I made the critical mistake of pushing myself to the breaking point physically, in the course of my training.

Somewhere along the line, I lost sight of the importance of balancing intense workouts with regular rest. I ended up with what's called Over-Training Syndrome.

Basically, it triggered a physical meltdown. It started with Tinnitus and Insomnia. To this day, some 17 years later, I have one ear that still rings and I take sleeping pills. It progressed to Colitis and then, all the symptoms of Fibromyalgia. My distance vision became blurry, and I had to get glasses. The absolute worst symptom of all is chronic fatigue. I was a dedicated endurance athlete for almost 30 years and now, I'm tired all the time. It ended my career.

Although I won't be racing anymore, I refuse to give in. I began running again even though it was very challenging. Just running for ten minutes was difficult, but I persisted. I ran for an hour the day that I began this chapter. Three days before that, I ran for 90 minutes. I'll walk 20 blocks to go for coffee. It's a long way from the four and five hour runs I used to do with ease. The important thing is that I'm doing what works for me under the current circumstances.

Doing the best you can is all that anyone can ask if you're battling sickness. Do whatever you can within the limits of your ability. You don't have to keep up with everyone else. If you can't run, then walk. If you can't walk, then swim. If you go to an aerobics class, don't worry about what the twenty-five year old at the front of the class is doing.

If you feel better walking or running in private, get a treadmill. If you feel self-conscious at aerobics class, get a DVD and do aerobics in your living room. Do whatever it takes to stay fit, and you'll improve your quality of life and longevity.

Most of all, your self-esteem will be enhanced with the knowledge that you didn't give in and are fighting the good fight no matter what.

CHAPTER NINE

THE AEROBICS ADVANTAGE

Aerobics is defined as a form of physical exercise that combines rhythmic aerobic exercise with stretching and strength training routines with the goal of improving all elements of fitness (flexibility, muscular strength, and cardio-vascular fitness).

Aerobics usually involves exercising at a low intensity for a long period of time at anywhere between 60 to 80 percent of maximum heart rate.

Although, it's roots were established way back in the 1960's when aerobics was developed by Dr. Kenneth H. Cooper, it really began to hit the mainstream in the mid-1980's.

Today, aerobics is still going strong and comes in many different forms.

AQUASIZE

Aquasize is also known as water aerobics and is often described as traditional aerobics without the impact.

Many seniors prefer aquasize because the buoyancy provided by being waist-deep in water takes away much of the impact on bones, joints, and muscles. The water adds pressure to the body which in turn, eases stress on joints, internal organs, and the heart.

Aquasize is also a great choice for seniors who want to ease their way into exercising. It has low impact, and decreases cardio and joint stress. At the same time, it improves endurance and lower and upper body strength.

Doctors will often recommend aquasize to senior patients who are overweight to ease the impact on joints. Seniors who suffer from osteoarthritis, knee and hip injury, or inflammatory diseases might also find out that aquasize is the perfect exercise for them.

Most of all, aquasize is a great way to instill social interaction into your exercise program. I would often watch seniors taking part in aquasize in an adjacent pool when I was swim training.

One thing that really struck me is that they always seemed to be smiling and having a great time.

JAZZERCISE

Jazzercise is a dance-based cardiovascular workout. It's for everyone regardless of age. In a way, it combines Pilates, yoga, strength training, and stretching.

A regular session might last a full hour, and include a warm-up and cool-down.

As a rule, current dance tunes is the music of choice, and the cardiovascular portion of the session is followed by strength training with small weights or tubes.

For seniors with time constraints, jazzercise is a great way to work on cardio, strength, and stretching all at the same time. It also compliments walking, running, swimming, or resistance training.

Many advocates of jazzercise claim to sleep sounder, have much more energy, and fewer headaches as well as the obvious benefits of increasing strength and flexibility.

ZUMBA

Just hearing the name zumba is often enough to scare off seniors.

When zumba first became a registered trademark in 2001, the workout sessions were considered very high intensity. Some people were of the opinion that you had to be in great shape just to join a class in order to survive the sessions.

Perhaps, it was the choice of music that gave the impression of high intensity. The music is a mixture of Latin and Rock, and the dance steps originated from salsa, calypso, reggae, merengue, tango, mambo, samba, and cha-cha.

I had a table at an expo once where I was doing book signings, and there was a zumba demonstration by an exercise class. I was amazed at how high the intensity level was, and how the primal beat of the music made you want to jump in and join them.

The great news for seniors is that Zumba Gold has been created just for them.

The intensity is toned down, but the excitement and liveliness of the upbeat music remains.

Zumba instructor, Claire Hadley, had this to say at the beginning of her Zumba Gold class for seniors...

"It doesn't matter if you start out on the wrong foot. And, if you swing the wrong arm and knock your neighbour over, just pick her up, dust her off and keep on moving! The main thing is to enjoy yourselves."

CHAPTER TEN

THE DIET DILEMMA

I've had the opportunity over the years to experiment with a number of different diet regimens. As an endurance athlete, I was trying to find the key to fueling my body so I could withstand intense training, and promote recovery so I could do it all over again. I also wanted to be able to perform at my best come race day.

I can't help but shake my head when I see all books that preach how complex carbohydrates are bad for you. The books are filled with page after page of nutritional hocus-pocus on the evils of carbohydrates, and the benefits of eating a diet consisting of mostly fat and protein.

There's no shortage of experts who claim that carbohydrates are responsible for the obesity epidemic sweeping across North America.

There are many Canadian health professionals who blame the Canadian Food Guide for the increase of obesity in Canada. In part, they're correct. Here's a look at the average recommended servings for adults according to the food guide.

7-8 vegetables and fruit

6-7 grain products

2 milk and alternatives

2 meat and alternatives

30 - 45 ml (2 to 3 Tbsp) of unsaturated oils and fats

It looks to be a recommended diet consisting of about 50% carbohydrates, but there's something missing from this equation. There's no allowance for level of fitness.

If a person has a sedentary job, and shuns exercising on a regular basis, they most likely would gain weight using this guide. They could indeed become obese. By the same token, the person who is fit and active would be fine following this guide.

The calories we consume in the form of complex carbohydrates, protein, and fat all have value and all serve a specific function in the maintenance of our bodies. Protein is needed to build muscle, complex carbohydrates is converted to glycogen for fuel, and high quality fats lower bad cholesterol, maintain healthy skin, and provide an additional source of fuel.

Once you wade through all the hocus-pocus about dieting and the evils of specific food choices, it really comes down to a simple formula.

If you are inactive, excess calories not needed to maintain your body according to your lifestyle will be converted to fat.

It doesn't matter if those calories come in the form of carbohydrates, protein or fat, any excess calories consumed will be stored away in fat cells that continue to grow larger. Normally, that fat first forms around the waist where it's easily accessible in the event that it's needed, and it spreads upwards and downwards from there. Basically, the body stores excess calories away for future use because that's the message it's being sent.

It seems to follow that there is one irrevocable truth that's likely the secret to weight gain.

If a person consumes more calories than they burn, they will gain weight.

It's not a mystery that you will lose weight if you eat nothing but quality fat and protein, and avoid simple and complex carbohydrates. In a nutshell, complex means no pasta, breads, rice, cereals, potatoes, or yams. Simple means no cake, cookies, pies, candy, fruit, or donuts. Well, you get the picture. Not only are you cutting back on calories, you're also cutting back on the glucose that's created when the body assimilates complex carbohydrates.

This is all very well, but just don't attempt any sort of physical activity that involves endurance because without sufficient glucose stores, you'll likely run out of gas. I experimented with this myself during the height of my athletic career, and the following is what I discovered through trial and error.

For a month, I went on a diet that consisted of mainly protein and fat with little in the way of carbohydrates. Then I entered a 10k race. I'd done the same race the year before and finished the 10k distance in just over 38 minutes. When the gun went off for the carbohydrate-free race, I knew I was in trouble after about 100 meters. I had a dramatic lack of energy. It took me five minutes longer to finish the race than it did the year before. That's a lifetime over that distance. It was glaringly obvious to me that complex carbohydrates were essential as a source of fuel for extended sessions of physical activity.

Here's another example.

When I was in the midst of my marathon career, another runner introduced me to a race diet that had become somewhat of a fad. It was called the carbohydrate depletion/loading diet. If the marathon was on a Sunday, you would begin the diet on the Sunday before.

Sunday, Monday, Tuesday, and Wednesday, the goal was to eat no carbohydrates at all. All that was allowed was protein and fat. Each one of those days, you ran an hour or so to ensure you used up all the glycogen stores still in your body. By not eating any carbohydrates, no glucose was created and by Wednesday, I was running on empty. By then, I could only run for ten minutes or so. I felt like death.

The second part of the diet from Thursday morning until race day was the carbohydrate loading phase. For the three days before the race, I ate every carbohydrate in sight. I loaded up on bread, pasta, potatoes, and brown rice. I could literally feel the energy surge back into my body. The idea of the diet was to mimic the late stages of the marathon where most runners use up their glycogen stores and hit the wall.

This diet faded away over the years because many runners found the depletion stage too difficult and detrimental to their health and wellbeing. Today most runners just do the carbohydrate loading part of this controversial diet.

If you follow one of the many diets that encourage you to eat mostly fat and protein and no carbohydrates, they are basically prompting you to adopt the carbohydrate depletion diet that I just described. If you stick with this for a month, I pretty much guarantee you'll lose weight. As a matter of fact, after a week, you'll probably lose weight.

The problem is that most people just can't do it. It's too hard. It takes too much discipline, and it makes you feel like crap. So they keep looking for the perfect diet that will let them eat some of the good stuff.

Here's what I deduced from all this.

Complex carbohydrates, protein, and fat all have a role to play, and should all be a part of the average person's diet. The key is to adjust the formula to your individual needs.

If you want to lose weight, the less complex carbohydrates you eat, the faster you will lose. That part is true. Just don't try and run ten miles because you won't have much energy.

If you're an endurance athlete, it would make sense to increase the amount of calories that come from complex carbohydrates. If you're a weight lifter, it would make sense to decrease the carbohydrates, and increase fat and protein to promote muscle growth.

I was training at a very intense level when I was entering Ironman Triathlon races. The race consisted of a 2.4-mile swim, a 112-mile bike, and a 26.2-mile marathon, all done one after the other. It was not unusual to swim two miles in training, and follow it up with a three hour bike training ride or two hour run. I was training six days a week, and working fulltime at a physically demanding job.

What I really needed at the time was the perfect diet to compliment the demands I was making in my body. I found it one day when someone handed me a book called Eat To Win.

It was written by a Dr. Robert Haas, and he claimed that athletes should increase their complex carbohydrate intake relative to their sport. One of his converts was tennis star Martina Navratilova. She was eating a diet of about 60% complex carbohydrates.

Dr. Haas claimed that his diet would improve endurance. Navratilova went on to beat top tennis stars that were half her age. She simply wore them down with her amazing endurance.

Over the years, I've often wondered if the *experts* who write on the evils of carbohydrates have ever tested their diets on the field of battle? Did they take their protein and fat only diet and attempt to run a marathon or do any type of extended physical exercise requiring stores of glycogen for fuel? Probably not.

Dr. Hass actually did, and was an established athlete who embraced distance running because of the endurance his own diet provided him with. That was reason enough for me to give his Eat to Win Diet a try.

I bought into the diet completely. Because of the training load I had, I was eating about 75% carbohydrates. That left 15% for protein and 10%

fat. I ate tons of pasta, brown rice, whole wheat bread and bagels, oatmeal, and potatoes. My main source of fat was extra virgin olive oil, coconut oil, and fish.

Tuna, white chicken, skim milk, low fat cottage cheese, and occasional lean beef provided most of the protein. The diet did not include simple carbohydrates like cake, cookies, ice cream, or any of those other sweet treats.

The Haas theory was that the complex carbohydrates were the high octane fuel that's burned in the fire of clean burning, high quality fat.

After one year on the diet, my race weight was 150 pounds just as it was 17 years prior when I first began running. In other words, despite all those carbohydrates I was eating, I didn't gain any weight.

If I'd eaten the same amount of carbohydrates for a year while sitting on the couch, I probably would've weighed 250 pounds or more.

In the Ironman race I was training for, I set new personal bests in the swim, bike, and run. I also set a new personal mark of 2:54 for the marathon. I was running 10K races in under 36 minutes. It was an amazing diet for my purposes.

Even today, at 68 years old, I balance my diet according to how physically active I am. I've found out that I can actually manipulate my weight whenever I want by altering the percentages of carbohydrates, protein, and fat I consume.

I've been running more a bit lately, so I've incorporated more complex carbohydrates into my diet. This morning, I ran for an hour and when I got home and weighed myself, I was 148 pounds. So, over the course of 40 years, my weight is basically exactly the same.

If I head down to Vegas or go on a cruise, all bets are off. I eat all the simple carbohydrates I normally avoid. I love ice cream, chocolate cake, and all those amazing cruise ship deserts and high end Vegas casino buffet treats. Most of the time, I'll come home, and will have gained six or seven pounds.

For three weeks, I'll go on the magical protein and fat only diet with no carbohydrates. During that three week period, I don't bother weighing myself and don't do any distance training as I have little energy. After about 20 days or so, I get back on the scale and sure enough I'm back to 150 pounds.

Probably a good starting point for today's senior is a diet of about 40% carbohydrates, 30% protein, and 30% fat. Make adjustments according to your lifestyle.

If you have a lot of weight to lose, eat a lower percentage of carbohydrates. If you really want to lose weight fast, don't eat any carbohydrates and focus on fat and protein until you get to your ideal weight.

If you're exercising on a regular basis, increase your complex carbohydrate intake to perhaps, 50%. If you're going all out and training for a marathon, increase it even more because as I explained above, you're burning carbohydrates for fuel in your training.

The calorie breakdown for someone aerobic exercising (walking, running, swimming, biking) on a regular basis might look like this:

25% protein, 25% fat, 50% carbohydrates. These are pretty much the Canada Food Guide recommendations. It makes sense for those exercising on a daily basis, but not so much if one is living a sedentary lifestyle. As the experts claim, it could lead to obesity.

If you decide you want to get stronger and get serious about resistance training, increase your fat and protein intake, and decrease your carbohydrate calories. You'll need the extra protein to rebuild new, stronger muscles.

The calorie breakdown for someone doing resistance training on a regular basis might look like this:

40% protein, 30% fat, 30% carbohydrates.

Of course everyone has a different metabolism, and the key is to experiment in order to find what works best for you. Keep close track of your weight and what you're eating on a daily basis as you do your exercise of choice.

There are also those who are diet-restricted because of health reasons. Regardless of the diet one is restricted to, it's often still possible to work out an ideal calorie intake.

For example, gluten free diets are currently center-stage on the fad diet merry-go-round.

A gluten free diet is essential for people suffering from Celiac Disease. I understand that part, but came across a startling statistic the other day. About forty percent of people on a gluten free diet don't have Celiac Disease.

They just decided it was a healthier diet. More to the point, they probably got stampeded by the so-called experts who claim that wheat is the root to all diet evil.

Strangely enough, there are more and more studies popping up in recent years that suggest people who do not have celiac disease should not be encouraged to go on a gluten free diet.

According to Dr, Leffer of Harvard Health..

"Gluten free products are not fortified with vitamins. This can create a problem. Whole wheat is also a major source of dietary fiber. Take away whole wheat and the problem gets worse."

After looking into what foods are allowed on a gluten-free diet, I have to say that personally, I wouldn't really find it all that restrictive. It would be a simple matter of adding important essential vitamins that are not available in gluten free products.

I suppose everyone would be impacted differently depending on what their usual food choices were before being restricted to a gluten-free diet.

Fruit, vegetables, meat, fish, dairy, eggs, beans, olive oil, and coconut oil are allowed.

Beans, egg whites, skim milk, and occasional, lean meat were my main sources of protein while training. Olive oil, coconut oil, and fish were my favorite high quality fats.

Brown rice, potatoes, and gluten-free oatmeal are also allowed. To this day, these three foods are among my top choices for complex carbohydrate power food. In a pinch, brown rice gluten free spaghetti by Lundberg would be an alternative choice for a pasta fix.

The only foods I would really miss would be whole wheat bread and bagels.

I have seldom eaten simple carbohydrates for most of my adult life because I was always in training. As a result, I wouldn't miss cookies, pies, cakes, muffins, crackers, or sweets of any kind for that matter. I would only eat these foods on occasion if I broke training for a week or two while on vacation.

Diets mean different things to different people. Everyone eats the way they do for a reason. Some people are restricted because of medical conditions, some have no self-control and eat anything, and some have strict diets like mine that are self-imposed for any number of reasons.

The one constant that I discovered over the years is that much like exercising, the body reacts to the signals it receives from the food we eat.

More is not better. The body takes only what's necessary to sustain the way we each live our lives. It takes all the extra calories we consume and converts them to fat.

We are all masters of our own body. Of course there are medical exceptions, but for the most part, we all have the power to dictate the physical transformation our body goes through on a daily basis.

Give your body the necessary resources it needs through optimum diet and regular exercise to maintain the highest level of efficiency, and you'll be amazed at the results.

CHAPTER ELEVEN

FOOD FOR THOUGHT

I'm in my 48th year in the grocery business.

It seems like just yesterday when Kraft Dinner would go on sale 10 for a dollar. You could buy a whole case of 48 for $4.80. I know because we did it when I shared a big old house with about four other guys just off the Red Mile, in Calgary.

I was about 19 years old and back then, KD, beans, and beer were some of the staples that we were seldom without. Today, you might get three or four boxes of Kraft Dinner for $4.80.

I remember those days when nobody really knew what yogurt was. It came in plain only, and would often just sit on the shelf until it reached its best before date. We'd throw it out and start over with a new batch. Along the way, something happened. I guess somebody said it was good for you, and the yogurt sections on the dairy shelves became wider and wider.

Eventually, someone decided that adding a bit of fruit flavor would be just the ticket. Soon, the plain yogurt that was good for you became sugar bombs, not unlike ice cream. The rest is history. Dozens of companies have jumped on the bandwagon and now, some yogurt sections are over 20 feet wide and five shelves high.

The produce department was where I spent a lot of my time over the years. As July arrived, B.C. Bing Cherries would go on sale for 59 cents a pound. Shortly after that, when corn season arrived, you could pick up a dozen for 69 cents.

I remember when the very first case of kiwi fruit made its appearance, when I was a Produce Manager in Toronto. Nobody knew what the Hell those little furry brown things were. We did everything but poke them with a stick, trying to figure out what they were. We put them on display, and threw them out about five days later. The customers were as mystified as we were.

It really looked like kiwi fruit would never make it in the marketplace. Then I guess they started to advertise that they were good for you too. One kiwi fruit had as much potassium as a banana they claimed. Within a couple of years, we were ordering 10 cases at a time. Sometimes, they would go on special five for a dollar, and we would order a lot more.

We used to sell this amazing bacon called Tulip. It was from Denmark, and it came in a red and white can. The bacon was wrapped in wax paper and folded over in half to fit into the tall can. It was the best bacon I ever tasted. It usually sold for around 69 cents. It was perfect to take camping. The regular bacon in the meat department was often on sale for around 89 cents. You could buy a good-sized cross-rib roast or pork roast for a few dollars. Wieners were around 59 cents a package.

Today, the average prices for these products sure have changed. The average price for bacon in 2017 is about $5.99, and it goes up to $7.99. That's not for a pound either. A package of bacon has been down-sized to 375 grams.

As if we wouldn't notice.

That good-sized cross-rib roast would now set you back over $30 and wieners, the poor man's food, have quadrupled in price.

This is what they mean when they talk about increase in cost of living. So, what's a senior to do once they're retired and on a fixed income? For most seniors, food is one of their biggest expenses. Apparently, people eat less as they age. I don't really buy into that completely.

If a senior adopts a lifestyle that includes regular exercise, a proper balance of carbohydrates, protein, and fat is important. As a rule, the more you exercise, the more you'll eat. After all, food is your source of fuel. The trick is to find alternate, less expensive food choices that can still ensure a healthy diet.

I sort of just shake my head when I walk through supermarket meat aisles. The odd time I'll buy chicken or lean ground beef if it's on sale. Even though I live alone, I'll often buy a turkey or two during the Easter, Christmas, or Thanksgiving holiday. I almost always find them at about .99 a pound for the 8-10 pound variety because it's such a competitive market for turkeys during the holidays.

Often, turkeys are used as loss leaders to draw people into the store. I cook them at any time of the year, and create about a dozen frozen meals. I just refuse to pay the sky high prices they're asking for meat these days. Besides that, I never did eat a lot of meat to begin with.

When I was a highly competitive athlete, my main sources of protein were 2% cottage cheese, skim milk, black beans, egg whites, canned tuna, sardines, and salmon. A single 170g can of tuna has about 15 grams of protein. A 540g can of black beans has 13 grams of protein. Both of these can be purchased for as low as $1.00 if you're willing to wait for them to go on sale. Canned salmon and the dairy products I mentioned can be pricey, but they're a bargain compared to buying meat as your main source of protein.

I rinse black beans and use them in omelettes and salads all the time. Of course you can use tuna or salmon in a salad or sandwich, or eat it right out of the can.

I know of weight lifters who eat three or four cans of tuna a day because they need the protein to rebuild muscles.

Pasta, rice, potatoes, and whole wheat bread are excellent choices for complex carbohydrates. Oatmeal, puffed wheat, and shredded wheat are the only cereals I eat as none of these have sugar and salt added. If you look at the ingredients on the box, it says wheat or oats and nothing else. When I have oatmeal, I add in raisins, banana (the only two fruits I ate during training) skim milk, and top it off with cinnamon. You can always add a sweetener or a bit of brown sugar for a treat. I call it oatmeal supreme. The best part about oatmeal is that the price is still very reasonable. I suggest buying the biggest bag when they're on sale.

Fat is present in a lot of these foods in differing amounts, but I use extra virgin olive oil on a daily basis to ensure I get a quality fat. I have a salad pretty much every day. The salad contains the vegetables that were the best price when I last shopped.

My dressing is olive oil and red wine vinegar (or balsamic vinegar). Personally, I never buy salad dressings off the shelf.

Another excellent option for quality fat is virgin coconut oil. You can use it as a replacement in any of your cooking and baking in a recipe that calls for margarine or butter.

When I was training, I also put coconut oil in my oatmeal and pasta. Olive oil and coconut oil are what I call big ticket items when it comes to groceries. The way I rationalize it is that I'm not buying that $20 steak or $40 roast, and in its place, I'm buying these healthy fats instead.

It's no contest.

In the past, many of the biggest grocery chains adopted the one-stop-shopping policy. Instead of just selling food, they sold non-food items that had nothing to do with groceries. Some stores even had mini-banks, and almost all have delicatessens and pharmacies.

The idea was that customers could buy everything they needed without going to a competitor. It wasn't at all unusual to see lawn chairs, patio tables, and sleeping bags in your local supermarket. In the last decade or so, major drug store chains began selling increased amounts of food products.

Now, Wal-Mart has also gone into the grocery business big time. So, basically all these retailers are trying to be all things to all people. It has caused a shift in the way the wise consumer shops.

These days, savvy consumers buy specific groceries from the store that has the best price as they vary so much from store to store. For example, they might buy meat in one store, produce in another, and canned goods down the street. Basically, there's a grocery price war going on every week. Whenever possible, seniors should take advantage of this. In most cities, you don't have to travel that far to visit four different retail locations.

When grocery stores run their weekly ads, they tend to go in about a 4-6 week cycle. It would be smart to buy enough of a product that's on sale to last you until it goes on sale again.

Let me give you an example. At one store I shop at, 540g cans of black beans, pinto beans, kidney beans, and usually, pork and beans, go on sale about every six weeks at a great price of 10/$1.00. I buy enough to last me until the next sale.

Why not?

Why would I go back the next week and pay the regular price of $1.69 or more? If it's a non-perishable item that you know you're going to use, why not stock up? Your fridge freezer should also be full of frozen food you bought on sale.

I don't hesitate at all to buy house brand products. In most cases, they're as good, and sometimes, better than the big name national brands that cost much more.

I just have to tell you about this App I came across. I just love it. It's a free App called Flipp. It has the current flyers for every supermarket in your city. The best part is that you can search for a particular item. It will show you the different prices for that product in all the different stores.

I always use it for things like olive oil and coffee that are fairly expensive. If it shows you a store that has olive oil on sale for $7.99, why would you pay $10.99 or more somewhere else? I always check out the Flipp App before shopping for the more expensive items.

If seniors pay attention to ongoing price shifts in grocery retail, they can probably cut 25% or more from their monthly food bill.

CHAPTER TWELVE

IS IT TIME TO RETIRE?

Retiring can be quite a shock to the system. After working for 40 or 50 years, it's quite an adjustment when it's all over and everything just stops. There's no more alarms to wake up to, and no traffic jams to fight.

At first, retirement might seem great. Finances won't be a problem because you've been very methodical about squirreling money away when the paychecks stop coming in. You have plans for travelling all over the place, and doing those renovations around the house.

That's a great plan, but what do you do when you are tired of airport security lineups, cruise ship buffets, and crowded Vegas sidewalks? You've got the nest all fixed up the way you want it, and you've run out of things to do around the house. So what's left? Shouldn't all that money you saved buy you happiness?

Unfortunately, the main pastime after retirement seems to be watching television...a lot of television.

Seniors 55 and up spend almost 40 hours a week watching T.V. That average number climbs substantially at 65 years of age to over 50 hours. In the USA, it's estimated that African Americans watch 218 hours of T.V. a month.

As people age, they tend to gravitate to television as a lifeline. They might feel useless and ignored out in the real world.

Remember when we were young and old people always got in the way? They drove too slow, and they walked too slow. It took them forever to decide what to buy from the grocery shelf, and they blocked the aisle with their shopping cart. When they got to the check-stand, they fumbled around for their money or took four tries to enter their debit card PIN number at the check-stand.

Now it's our turn.

As seniors slow down, they become more and more aware of the negativity toward them out in the world. They sense the lack of compassion, and seek solace in front of the television.

A decade ago, cartoonist Jules Feiffer drew a bead on the problem, penning a strip in which an older man sits talking to his TV.

"No one loves me," the man says, and the TV responds, "I love you."

Each time the man complains that he has no one to take care of him, to give to him, or to be his friend, the TV assures him that he is not alone. It's a sad commentary of the times when a television becomes a senior's best friend.

If a senior is healthy and enjoys the work they do, it could be a good idea to put off retiring. This would be especially beneficial if one is single with no pressing plans for retirement, or if retirement financial goals haven't been reached yet.

Really, what's another five years if you're in good health? People are living longer and longer all the time. Working until the age 70, and sometimes longer, is becoming common-place.

According to Stats Canada in 2015, there were 5,780,900 Canadians over 65. There were

5,749,400 Canadians under 15. One of the main reasons why older Canadians are outpacing the younger ones is that people are living a lot longer than they used to.

Great strides have been made in the world of medicine in the past couple of decades. Many diseases that were at one time deadly can now be treated. Even if a person will never be completely free of a particular disease, there are prescription medicines that can extend their lives for years or even decades. As a result, a senior in good health could work until 70, and still have a couple of decades to enjoy retirement.

If you've ever taken a two week holiday and just stayed around the house, you'll have some idea just how much time you'll have on your hands when you have 52 weeks of work free bliss. If you're single, you'll have even more free time because there's nobody else around to light a fire under you to do things.

I personally made the decision to continue working on a part-time basis once I reached 65. I realized that if I collected my CPP, OAS, and company pension, and worked three days a week instead of five, my income was pretty well exactly the same.

The only difference now is that I just work three days and have four days off per week. It was a no-brainer.

Working part-time might be a strategy for seniors to consider. Of course it has to be possible with their particular job. Quitting work cold turkey can be stressful, and working part-time for a while can ease the transition into retirement.

Even just being home a couple of extra days every week provides a better understanding of just how much free time you'll end up with when you retire for good.

So, what can you do with all that spare time when you do eventually retire? Surely, there are more productive, satisfying, and selfless goals besides watching T.V, gaining weight, and watching your health deteriorate.

You bet there are! You're capable of so much more than you give yourself credit for. All you have to do is believe in yourself, and think outside of the box a little. Retirement shouldn't be depressing and frightening.

It should be the beginning of the best years of your life.

CHAPTER THIRTEEN

GOLDEN VOLUNTEERS

Volunteers are the lifeblood of many organizations. The amount and variety of volunteer positions in any city anywhere in the world are abundant. The trick is to find the volunteer niche that's perfect for you because it's not just your time that's valuable. It's your passion, skill, and knowledge that's priceless as well.

If you have love for animals, then volunteering at the local Zoo or Humane Society (SPCA) might just be the perfect fit. There are dozens of positions animal shelters need filled, but you may have to go on a waiting list as they are snapped up pretty quick. Lots of people want to work with kittens and puppies.

If you want to work with kids, check out the local Boys and girls Club organization. They'll most likely have a variety of positions available. Just out of curiosity, I did a Google search for volunteer positions with the Boys and Girls Clubs of Calgary, because that's where I live. They had over 20 volunteer positions available.

The one that really intrigued me was assistant cook at their summer camp. They were looking for someone with a cooking background to spend about two summer months of 2017 in their wilderness camp, helping to feed around 100 kids and staff. Someone who has the necessary skills, enjoys kids, and has a love for the great outdoors would probably really enjoy this.

It just goes to show that there are some very unique volunteer opportunities out there.

Are you a carpenter, plumber, painter, or electrician by trade? Habitat for Humanity is always looking for volunteers, and what a great way to put your skills to work. It's not necessary to be skilled in a trade to volunteer for this great cause. Enthusiasm and a willingness to help those less fortunate are all you really need.

Most likely, there's a Habitat home being built in or around your city. Currently, they have about 65,000 volunteers who help build homes across Canada. There are also opportunities to take part in the Global Village program. You could find yourself making a trip to India, Thailand, Costa Rica, or any number of countries in need of affordable housing. If interested, it's just a matter of contacting the nearest of 58 affiliates located across the country.

Do you have love for books? Public libraries are always looking for volunteers to help with computer technology, getting reading material to shut in seniors, and exposing youth to the joy of reading.

Perhaps, The Red Cross would be more to your liking. The Red Cross is always right there when disaster strikes, to provide assistance to those in need. As with many organizations, potential volunteers would have to apply, submit references, and for some positions dealing with vulnerable persons, submit to additional screening. You could be a part of the largest humanitarian organization in the world.

I had first-hand experience with the crucial role the Red Cross plays in the event of natural disasters when I was flooded out of my home on two different occasions. When all seems lost, it's truly uplifting to see volunteers wearing the Red Cross armband coming to your aid. It's truly an excellent organization, and one you would surely be proud to be part of.

Food Banks are always in need of people willing to donate their time. They need help on the trucks with food pick up, sorting and assembly lines, baby room, special events, and people to take phone calls, and to interview walk ins. It docsn't matter what city you live in, there will always be people in need of food, to help them through difficult times. This means there will always be a need of volunteers to make it happen.

Every city has seniors who need help with a variety of chores they are unable to manage on their own. They need help with meals, mowing lawns, clearing snow, and perhaps filing, their income tax and other paper work.

There's something special about seniors helping seniors. Maybe it's because one day, it could be you who is in need of help. It's sort of like paying it forward in advance.

If you are so-inclined, there are some very emotionally and mentally demanding volunteer positions. For instance, I spent a year answering Distress Center phone calls from people who were in desperate situations. Like many other demanding volunteer positions, there is training involved to ensure you are able to handle any contingency.

Volunteers who work with children can have a huge impact on their lives. When someone goes out of their way to help a child in the formative days of their youth, that child will never forget it.

The Vancouver Boys Club was my second home during a turbulent childhood, and over 50 years later, I still remember every volunteer I crossed paths with. I remember their names and what they looked like. I remember the movies they took me to, the new sport they taught me, and how they were always there when I need someone to talk to.

Volunteering can leave a lasting impact, and is about much more than just filling in idle time. It's about making a difference to those most in need, and leaving a legacy that will be there long after you're gone.

CHAPTER FOURTEEN

BE YOUR OWN BOSS

"I was sixty-six years old. I still had to make a living. I looked at my social security check of 105 dollars and decided to use that to try to franchise my chicken recipe. Folks had always liked my chicken."

--Colonel Sanders

What an inspiring story. Colonel Sanders was 66 years old when he took matters into his own hands, and started his own business. I'm willing to bet that pretty much anyone who reads this book has at some point in their life, fantasized about opening their own business.

Maybe some of you made it a reality, but for most, it was a wistful dream that never saw the light of day. It was a bridge too far, a mountain too high.

You were younger then.

You had a business in mind that you were sure you could make work. It was something you had a passion for, but it was scary starting out so early in life by taking such a big gamble. What if you failed? You opted for the easy way out, and worked for someone else instead. It was easier to let the boss take all the risks. All you had to do was show up to work on time, punch in, do the job, and punch out. There was no risk involved. You picked up your paycheck like clockwork, week after week, and every year, took your well-earned vacation time.

But perhaps, behind the facade of contentment and job security, there was a lingering question that always sort of haunted you.

What if?

What if you had said damn the torpedoes and charged headfirst into the world of entrepreneurship? Where would you be now and how different would your life have been? As you collect your final paycheck and settle into retirement, maybe not much has changed. Maybe you still wonder, what if?

Who says you still can't live your dream? Who says it's too late to follow your passion? Chances are you're probably in a much better financial position now than you were when having your own business was a youthful dream.

You also have decades of worldly experience on your side, and have a better understanding of how business works. It's not too late to take your passion and run with it.

The good news is that today, there are other options besides a big financial outlay for a brick and mortar location. The era of the internet has opened up small business opportunities for thousands of budding entrepreneurs with a product to sell.

What's your passion?

Perhaps, you're skilled at making unique costume jewellery, or have a great idea for a healthy food product. There are several options for selling your wares online. You can open a store on your own website, or you can opt to sell your product through E-bay or Amazon. Your online business can be as big or as small as you want it to be.

Around the year 2000, a woman named Linda Lightman wanted to earn some extra money and decided to give E-bay a try. She began by selling stuff from her home that was no longer being used. She sold her sons old video games and then, progressed to clothes, shoes, and jewelry she no longer had use for.

Word got out and she started selling stuff for her friends. By 2006, she had 20 employees and had to buy a 5000 square foot office space. She had to increase her retail space four times over the years and by 2015, the new home for *Linda's Stuff* was 93,000 square feet.

Her income grew to a staggering twenty-five million dollars annually. Her husband became president of the company, and her son is Vice President of business development. Her husband, Fred, graduated from Columbia Law School, and her son spent two years working in investment banking in New York.

Of course her story is exceptional, but it does show that an online business can succeed. The beauty of the E-bay business model is that the initial financial outlay is minimal. You have a product to sell, somebody buys it, E-bay takes their cut and you ship it to the purchaser. Anybody can do that without even opening an E-bay storefront.

I once sold a racing bike for $1600 on E-bay. If the price is right, there's virtually a buyer for just about anything you can think of selling.

There are more benefits to selling a product online besides the financial ones. Let's say for instance, you have a passion for antiques, and you open an E-bay store and begin stocking it. You travel all over the city and nearby countryside, searching for hidden gems in estate auctions, obscure antique stores, and second hand shops. You buy something amazing for $20, and you just know it's worth way more.

What a great way to get out there and keep yourself busy with all that free time on your hands during retirement. While enjoying the thrill of the hunt, you get to see new places and meet tons of people along the way. It also helps keep you physically, emotionally, and mentally fit.

If you want to interact with people on a person-to-person basis as opposed to the anonymity of an internet business, there are several other options you might consider.

Using antiques as the same example, there's nothing stopping you from purchasing space at local flea markets, and showing off your amazing finds. Whether you bake the best pies or cookies for miles around, or have developed a new product, there will always be venues where you can test the market.

If you have a new product idea, and you want to see if there's a demand before committing to a brick and mortar retail, you might consider trade fairs. There are trade fairs for just about everything. I've been to automobile, outdoor recreation, sporting goods, and Home and Garden trade fairs just to name a few.

Whatever you decide, it's never too late to live your dream of owning your very own business. It doesn't have to be on a huge scale.

Start out small and see where it takes you.

CHAPTER FIFTEEN

WRITE WHAT YOU KNOW

There's no doubt in my mind that everyone has a book in them just waiting to see the light of day. Perhaps, there are those who wistfully think about writing a book but feel it's beyond them. They're convinced that writing books is a craft bestowed on the gifted few.

Maybe they feel qualified to write a book but can't seem to come up with a storyline. In other words, they're thinking more along the lines of writing fiction. It seems to me that a good first step to take in the world of writing is to write what you know. In other words, write a non-fiction book.

About 11 years ago, I was a million miles away from writing a book.

My main concern at the time was figuring out how to use a computer, and dealing with the complexity of building a website. I was in my 50's, and completely out of the loop when it came to computers, but I had something to say.

I'd learned a lot about endurance sports and the Ironman Triathlon in general, after 30 years of training and racing. My goal was to build a website so I could share what I'd learned with others who were just starting out in the sport of triathlon.

So that's what I did.

Once I had the website built, I just kept posting articles about all the different aspects of endurance training and racing. The focus was on the Ironman Triathlon in particular because that's what I knew best. It had taken me years of experimenting to learn about proper nutrition, best training practices, and how to approach race day when it arrived. Mostly, what I did was tell people the mistakes I made over the years, and how I eventually overcame them.

I was certain the information I shared had the potential to inform, inspire, and motivate my visitors to become more than they ever thought possible. Then one day, about a year after my website, Ironstruck.com was up and running, something remarkable happened that would change my life.

I received an email from a triathlete on the other side of the world. He and his twin brother were preparing to compete in Ironman South Africa that was set to take place in the City of Port Elizabeth the following week. He said, "we love your website and we're printing off a lot of the articles to take to the race with us."

He was referring to the information I'd written about what happens the days leading up to the race, the eve of the race, and the morning of the race. Basically, what I'd written on my website walked those new to the Ironman through the whole process of how to be best prepared when the gun went off on race morning.

Then he wrote these magical six words that I will never forget.....

"Why don't you write a book?"

I just looked at the computer screen for about 30 seconds after reading those words, and it hit me that he was exactly right. Why not indeed? Why not put everything I had learned over the years into a book that people could refer to all during the training year and then, take to the race with them?

What a great idea.

Even though I had no idea how to actually put a book together, it really turned out to be easier than

I thought. These days, there are thousands of resources on the internet that can help you create the actual book, but you are the only one who can write what's in your heart and mind. You just have to believe in yourself, and be brave enough to write those first few words.

If I could write a book back then, despite my misgivings about being in over my head, I have no doubt that you can as well. Once the words start to flow, it's like the floodgates have opened. All that knowledge you have about whatever your passion is can't wait to get out.

You may think your passion is obscure but it's almost a certainty there will be many others somewhere in the world with the same interest who will be anxious to read what you have to say.

Keep in mind that you can create an E-book as well as a hard copy. An E-book makes your book accessible to people on the other side of the world with a few clicks of a computer mouse.

The easiest way to write your non-fiction book about your passion is to imagine you're having coffee with someone, and they're asking you all these questions about your passion. So for example, they're asking you about roses because roses have been your passion for years, and you know so much about them. You have a plethora of information stored in your memory bank of all the things you did right and wrong when it came to growing roses.

Personally, I don't know a thing about roses, so I might ask you questions like this. Where did roses come from anyway? What are the different varieties of roses? Are there certain roses for certain climates? What colors do they come in? Do roses come from bulbs or seeds? When is the best time to plant? What is the best type of soil?

Okay, so you get my drift. Those could be the first seven chapters of your book about roses.

I don't know if chapters are even the right name, because in my first book, Ironstruck...the Ironman Triathlon Journey, I have 62 such topics listed on the contents page. They ranged in length from one page to three pages. Remember, someone needs answers to the questions concerning the passion you're writing about. It doesn't take 15 pages to answer a question.

Say what you have to say and go on to the next logical question that someone might ask. When you've answered all the relative questions you can possibly think of that might be of interest to your reader, your book is finished.

It really doesn't matter if you want to write about roses, restoring old cars, fly fishing, or making costume jewelry. To write a book, all you need is three main ingredients. You need passion, knowledge born of experience, and the willingness to share what you know.

You need passion because readers will feel it in your words as they read your book, and it will inspire and motivate them. It makes them feel more connected to you. It makes them want to succeed.

Knowledge born of experience is very powerful.

It's often more powerful than what's learned at an institute of higher learning. Readers will be moved by your description of the day as you were working in the garden and right before your eyes, a rosebud burst open into a brilliant red blossom. It flourished and grew in that same rosebush that had almost died the year before, and you figured out how to bring it back to life.

At that point, they could care less that you're not a trained Botanist.

It was much the same when I wrote in my first book. For example, after years of experimenting, I discovered whole wheat bagels with peanut butter and honey were the perfect race day fuel. They were easily cut into bagged portions to carry in a cycling jersey. This combination also provided the ideal balance of complex carbohydrates, fat, and protein, and easily assimilated by the body. It provide high octane fuel for the 112 mile bike, and 26.2 mile marathon. I went on to say that it was this same combination that enabled me to have my fastest Ironman bike and marathon times ever.

I'm almost certain that at this point, the reader didn't give a damn that I wasn't a licensed nutritionist, and didn't have a coaching licence.

They were reading what someone had actually learned through trial and error in the heat of battle. Experience will always be the best teacher and your readers will be moved by your willingness to share your failures as well as successes.

Not everyone has a willingness to share.

There are so many talented people in the world who keep a lifetime of experience and knowledge locked inside, and it often dies with them.

If you have a willingness to share your passion and knowledge, you could well change a person's life for the better. What a great legacy to leave behind. In your own way, you have the power to unselfishly make the world a better place to live.

So start writing that book.

You just might surprise yourself and one day, be sitting at the front of a major bookstore signing your work. Once you start writing, you might never stop. I doubted myself when I took on my first book and now, you're reading book number six.

Write what you know.

What a great way to spend your retirement.

CHAPTER SEVENTEEN

THE SINGLE SENIOR

The world is chock full of single seniors of all ages. It's well documented that scientific studies have found out that single seniors have a lower life expectancy rate. That has been known for a long time now.

Some seniors don't adapt well when they suddenly find themselves on their own due to the loss of a loved one. They have lost their main source of emotional and functional support.

It doesn't have to be that way.

There are seniors who have been single for quite a long time and manage quite well. Personally, I've been single for over 35 years. As the years pass by, one adapts to being on their own.

I could have chosen to just hang around home and drown in self-pity, but that wasn't the way I wanted to live my life. I decided that I was going to get out there, and make the most of the cards I'd been dealt. Soon, I was used to travelling alone and enjoyed the freedom that came with it.

A lot of people like to conform and refuse to travel unless they have someone to go with them. That's what most people do, isn't it?

This is especially true for women. Many women think it's taboo to travel alone. If they go on a cruise, they share a cabin with a stranger as opposed to being on their own. After all, what would people think if they were by themselves?

There's something special about travelling alone. It leaves you open to all possibilities and you just never know who will cross your path.

For example, there was this time in my travels when I met this beautiful single woman, who was a pharmacy manager from Switzerland, and spoke five languages. I was very impressed when she said she almost always travelled alone. She travelled all over the world and had no problem with it.

It was so amazing to meet her because she lived her life much like I did.

She was a free spirit and she was living life her way, not the way society thought she should. She had no hidden agenda, and was probably the most genuine person I ever met.

She reminds me of this quote.

"Your genuine action will explain itself...will explain your other genuine actions. Your conformity explains nothing" --Ralph Waldo Emmerson

Even though we both knew the limitations of the relationship that developed between us because we lived so far apart, it was still remarkable while it lasted.

She invited me to visit her in Nyon, the small town she lived in just outside of Geneva. If not for her, I probably never would've made it to Europe. It was something I never felt compelled to do, but I'm so glad that I finally did.

What a stunning country Switzerland is.

Several times, we met in the USA and would go on a cruise or to a land, stay on a beautiful Caribbean island together. It was exciting to set up itineraries that would have us meeting in Boston, New Orleans, or Miami as our jumping off point.

We both loved the island of Martinique, and I have this indelible image of her running beside me on snow white, powdery sand as the surf crashed in, and the sun was just rising over the Caribbean Sea.

I remember glancing over at her. She was so lithe, and ran as effortlessly as the early sunbeams shimmered in her long auburn hair. She was truly luminous.

One afternoon, we sat in an outdoor cafe having a drink. I looked at her, and she gave me this dazzling smile. Behind her, I could see the iridescent blue sea, and endless stretches of perfect white sand. As clear as day, I can remember thinking that I wished I could freeze that moment in time. I never wanted it to end.

But all things must end.

I wasn't really surprised when two years later, she emailed me to say she was marrying a Swiss doctor. I don't even know how she stayed single as long as she did. What an amazing woman.

I've often wondered...

What if I'd just stayed home and never got myself out into the world? I would've missed out on these truly special memories.

Yes, being single has its drawbacks. Sure, there are times when you feel lonely. But I realized a long time ago, that you have to get out there because you just never know what might happen.

It doesn't mean you have to go to some far off tropical destination. You could just as well connect with someone special at a community potluck dinner, or while volunteering your time for a worthy cause.

In many ways, we bring loneliness upon ourselves. It really doesn't matter if you're 50 or 70 or 80, if you don't make an effort to socialize, nothing is going to change.

Whether you hope to meet someone special or simply want to create amazing memories, you have to be willing to get out there. Be yourself, and not what you think people expect you to be.

It's the special memories we retain that can sustain us all the years of our life.

In general, I think things are really looking up for single seniors. In the past, it was difficult for seniors to physically impose on family and friends. The end result is, they were often left to their own devices.

I'm sure there are single seniors out there who's greatest fear is dying alone. They fear dying without anyone even knowing they passed away.

Times have certainly changed for the better, and there is no reason this has to happen.

If a senior wants to keep in touch with family or perhaps, meet a significant other, the world of social media is there for them. The high tech age is a reality, and it's here to stay.

Email, Twitter, Facebook, and Instagram are just a few unobtrusive ways for seniors to stay connected with the world outside their door.

All it really takes is to have someone contact you on a regular basis. All it takes these days is a simple phone message. How are you? Is everything ok? Is there anything you need?

The internet also opens up the possibility of connecting with someone on a dating site. There are some websites like ourtime.com that are specifically for seniors.

If you're a senior and you spot someone at one of these sites who interests you, why not arrange a meeting for coffee somewhere public?

Be sure to take care in how you word your ad. You don't want to turn off prospective suitors. For instance, an ad like this might not work in your favor.

Recent widow who has just buried fourth husband looking for someone to round out a six-unit plot. Dizziness, fainting, shortness of breath not a problem.

Even if you meet someone and don't hit it off as far as a lasting relationship, you may make a new friend. Eventually, you could build your own network of senior friends who look out for each other via social media.

The key is to find what makes you happy.

It might be as simple as regular coffee meetings with a group of friends. Once you have things to look forward to, being single isn't such a bad thing after all.

CHAPTER SEVENTEEN

ROAD WARRIORS

I'm sure many seniors are dreading the day when someone tells them they can no longer drive.

Being able to drive gives seniors independence, and a sense of control. The ability to drive makes it much easier to stay active on a social level. It also makes it more convenient for everyday tasks like doctor's appointments, grocery shopping, or perhaps, making it to your volunteer position.

Having to count on taxis and public transportation to get where you want to go can be extremely inconvenient and trying.

There are other ramifications besides losing your ability to drive from A to B behind the wheel of your own vehicle.

It can be depressing to be told you're simply too old to do something you've done all your life. You could begin to feel that it's just one more thing that pushes you to the back-burner of society into an old folk's home.

Maybe you're not ready to be relegated to the golden ghetto.

There are several health issues that can make being behind the wheel a dangerous proposition. These are some indicators that can signal the end of your driving days.

Something as simple as a stiff neck could take away the ability to check the blind spot while changing lanes. Weak arms can make it difficult to turn a steering wheel quickly in case of emergency. Sore, stiff legs can make simple functions like moving your foot from the gas to brake pedal more challenging.

Slowed reflexes could make merging into traffic or braking on time for pedestrians a hit or miss proposition.

It's no secret that heart disease and diabetes have been linked to seniors being involved in car accidents. There have also been studies that indicate seniors who have fallen are more likely to get into automobile accidents.

Falling indicates several physical issues including weak lower bodies, poor balance, and slow reaction time. On top of all that, as seniors age, there's normally a reduction in strength, flexibility, and coordination.

There are several ways you can extend your ability to drive.

As you age, being fit has a positive impact on just about every facet of your life, and driving is certainly no exception. Exercising on a regular basis has the potential to increase your ability to stay behind the wheel for years longer than the norm.

As discussed earlier, walking, running or swimming, or aerobics are good examples of physical activities that can improve upper and lower body strength, flexibility, and reaction time.

These are all functions critical to driving.

Resistance training can also increase leg, back, neck and shoulder strength. It's well worth the effort to exercise on a regular basis if it makes you a safer driver and keeps you on the road far into your senior years.

As much as you might like the current car you're driving, updating to a new model might also help you stay behind the wheel longer.

Here are just a few of the options new cars are coming with these days:

- Touch screen navigation GPS to help you get where you're going
- Backup camera
- Seat lumbar support
- Parking assistance. It's very cool to see a car parallel parking itself.
- Automatic emergency response system
- Some models even have grab bars to help you get in and out of the car.
- There are some cars that will automatically brake for in case of impending collision.
- Lane Departure Warnings will let you know if you're drifting out of your land while at speed.

It might be tough for some seniors to give up the car they're used to driving. There's the cost factor to consider as well. Not every senior will be able to afford to trade up to a new model. Seniors might also be scared off by all the new technology they'd have to learn, but most likely, there's someone in your life who could help you learn how everything works.

Anything you can do to allow yourself to drive longer is well worth the investment in time, effort, and money. Having independence is a wonderful thing, and you should hang on to it for as long as you can.

The more years you continue to drive, the closer you will be getting to the day when cars drive themselves. Google already has prototypes that have no steering wheel, and drive to a pre-set destination while the passenger relaxes in a seat.

The day is coming when this concept will be mainstream. What a plus it will be for seniors who are unable to drive. As unbelievable as it may seem, the day this becomes a reality is closer than you might think.

CHAPTER EIGHTEEN

GOOGLE IS YOUR FRIEND

Google is basically a window to the world and an amazing tool for finding answers to your question. I'm kind of surprised at how many people don't know how to make the most of it. I don't mean just seniors. For instance, I had a question from a visitor to my website. He said he was thirty and he was wondering what exercises were best for getting stronger leg muscles.

I typed this into Google search...*what exercises are best for getting stronger leg muscles?*

There were 36,500,000 answers to the question that popped up. I picked one that came complete with images and video, and sent the link to him. He sent a reply, "thanks! That's just what I needed." Go figure. I guess he didn't know how to use Google. I included some examples below for those of you who are unsure of how to get the most out of Google.

Type these into Google for charts on life expectancy. If you are interested in a particular year, be sure to add it into your search.

- Life expectancy statistics Canada or (specific year here)life expectancy statistics Canada
- USA life expectancy tables

If your questions don't have to be specific to where you live, there's no need to put your location in the search.

- Seniors and the benefits of running
- Seniors and walking for fitness
- Resistance training programs for seniors
- Benefits of resistance training for seniors
- Weight training programs for seniors
- Benefits of weight training for seniors
- Senior fitness after heart surgery

If you want to improve your chances of seeing images or videos, simply add them into your search. Keep in mind that you can put emphasis on a particular word in your search by using brackets. Most of your search results should contain the word in brackets.

- Senior weight training (videos)
- Senior weight training (images)

If you want to find information on buying a new or used treadmill, or volunteering for instance, always stipulate your city in the Google search. If you don't, you'll get Google results from all over the world.

The following search will give you options of companies that sell new treadmills. You'll most likely also get links to Kijiji ads, complete with new and used treadmills for sale in your city.

If you don't specify your city, you'll find treadmills for sale all over the world. For example,

- Treadmills for sale in (your city here)

You could also go straight to Kijiji but be sure to put your city in the search query as Kijiji is all over North America.

- Kijiji (put your city here) treadmills for sale

Looking for volunteer info?

- Volunteer info for Habitat for Humanity Canada

Here's how you narrow the same search for your part of the country:

- Volunteer info for Habitat for Humanity Southern Alberta (or your province of state)

Here's how you narrow it to your city:

- Volunteering with (put your city here) Red Cross
- Volunteering with (put your city) public library
- Volunteering with (put your city here) Human society
- Volunteering with (put your city here) food Bank

Looking for a dating site?

Be sure to stipulate Senior dating site in your city, province, or state. If you just type in dating sites, there are over 48 million hits to your query. If you stipulate senior and a particular city, there are just over two million hits.

- Dating for seniors (your city, province or state here)

Whatever you type in the search bar, the ten most relevant search results are normally on the first page that pops up. Sometimes, you can go two or three pages deep, and check out the top 30.

You could get 10 million hits from your query, but just concentrate on the first two few pages.

CAPTER NINETEEN

WORLD'S OLDEST PERSON

On April 12, 2017, the world's oldest living person passed away peacefully.

Emma Morano of Italy was 117 years, 137 days, and 16 hours old.

According to Wikipedia, the living person on record before Morano was Misao Okawa of Japan, who died on April 1, 2015 at the age of 117 years, 27 days.

Morano is the last person documented as being born in the 1800's. She was born in 1899.

It sure makes you wonder if some people are just fortunate to be blessed with longevity genes. Or is it more than that?

Those around her claimed Morano lived a simple life. She had no use for consumer goods over the course of her life, and left the world with little in the way of worldly possessions. There really wasn't much room in her small two room apartment anyway.

Of course many people wondered over the years what her secret to living so long was.

When she was a teenager, doctors told her she should move to a milder climate for health's sake. She moved to a small village called Verbania, in Piedmont. Maybe that was part of the reason.

She was diagnosed with anaemia when she was 20 years old, just after World War 1 ended. A doctor told her she should eat three eggs per day. So for the rest of her life, she ate 2 raw eggs and one egg in an omelet each day. It's estimated that she ate well over 100,000 eggs.

Never again will I feel guilty about the three egg omelets I enjoy several times a week.

She was not a big fan of fruit or vegetables, and ate very little of them. In the last few decades of her life, the mainstays of her diet was mostly eggs and cookies.

Really.

She was very independent, and cooked for herself until she was 112, and often enjoyed pasta with ground beef.

I really like this woman. I love pasta.

She quit eating meat when she heard it caused cancer. Chicken and eggs appeared to become her main source of protein in the last decade or so of her life.

She had an excellent work ethic, and had a job until she was 75.

It's also very interesting that after a failed marriage and separation in 1938, she never ever considered remarrying. She had an abusive husband, and decided she would never let that happen again.

As a result, she remained single and lived on her own for 79 years. She was 115 when she finally gave in, and had a live-in caregiver.

So what was her secret to longevity? Maybe it was in her genes after all. Her mother died at 91, and two of her sisters were over 100 when they died.

Remarkably, Morano was still about five years away from being the oldest person who ever lived. That distinction belongs to Jeanne Calment of France who lived to be 122.

It goes to show that it would serve us better to not consider ourselves old because we've reached a certain landmark age. It almost seems that old age is truly a irrelevant concept these days.

CHAPTER TWENTY

SENIORS ON THE MOVE

PEGGY ORR

Peggy Orr of Calgary, Alberta was still making her weekly forays to the dance floor of the Bowness Legion as she neared her 104th birthday. Her presence at the weekly gathering for seniors inspires others she crosses paths with to stay healthy and keep moving forward.

Perhaps, being born and growing up in a farm near Crossfield, where hard work was a way of life, instilled her with the same work ethic she had as a centenarian.

At 100 years old, Orr was still planting and caring for a garden and often going out for rides on her son's motorcycle.

Remarkably, up until 2016, Orr lived independently. When asked what the secret to her longevity was, she replied,

"Just keep busy, that's all, keep doing what you have to do."

GERTIE WILLIAMS

You're never too old to put your volunteer skills to work. At 102 years, old Gertie Williams was still teaching students how to read as part of the literacy program at the Belvedere Parkway School in Calgary, Alberta. Williams was part of the program as a volunteer when it began 20 years earlier. What a great way to stay active, and stay involved with the community.

As is often the case, Williams didn't slow down when she retired. She credits her longevity to getting out there and staying active into her senior years. She took up hiking, cross-country skiing, square dancing, and even belonged to a rifle club.

Williams has no plans to stop volunteering with kids because she believes it makes a difference. There's no doubt she has been a positive influence to hundreds of kids over the years.

OLIVE DODDS

At the age of 105, Olive Dodds was going strong as a 30 year volunteer with the Toronto East General Hospital. She was born before the Toronto Maple Leafs even existed. When she was five, she witnessed a German Zeppelin crash during the First World War.

The East General was at the very same hospital where Dodds had angioplasty surgery at age 92. She claims her key to longevity was having a positive outlook on life, and being happy and content. She never smoked, and drank very little. As a young nurse, she was used to working 12 hours at a time; so she was no stranger to hard work.

At 106, Olive Dodds was still on the move and maintaining her happy disposition.

Dodds is a perfect example that the way we approach each day on mental and emotional levels has a positive impact on quality of life as well as longevity.

CHARLES EUGSTER

Charles Eugster of Great Britain currently holds the world record for the indoor 60m and 200m, and outdoor 200m and 400m.

Not that many people have heard of him because he's 96 years old.

Eugster is also a body-builder, rower, public speaker, and entrepreneur.

What I found most interesting about his story is that he didn't begin weight training until he was 87. This is what he had to say about it.

"I was 87 and realized my body was deteriorating. I had a muffin-top waist and my muscles were getting weaker and weaker. I felt so old. But because I was so vain, I didn't like the idea of it at all. So I joined a body-building gym and employed a personal trainer who was a Mr. Universe to rebuild my body from scratch."

By challenging his body to improve and get stronger, Eugster reversed the aging process and feels more like he's 60, and in the process, it proved a beach body at 90 plus is possible.

Eugster claims to consume most of his calories in the form of protein and fat as opposed to carbohydrates.

This makes perfect sense as he focuses on weight lifting which require more protein to rebuild muscles. He also runs short distances and can get by with fewer complex carbohydrates.

ROBERT MARCHAND

Robert Marchand of France didn't begin to take cycling seriously until he was 68. At 100 years old, he set a record for distance covered on an indoor track in one hour. Two years later, he beat his own record. Marchand was far from done however. At the age of 105, a new category had to be established just for him. He cycled an amazing 14 miles in one hour. His cycling prowess is remarkable on several fronts.

First of all, Marchand has an amazing balance. We all know that you have to have balance in order to ride a bike. Imagine the balance required to ride at a good clip for one hour when you're 105 years old. He also has remarkable endurance.

Between the indoor cycle track records, he set two years apart, he biked long distances including a ride from Paris to Moscow. As expected, his diet consisted mainly of complex carbohydrates because he specialized in endurance events. As a rule, he never ate meat but did increase his protein intake during his more intensive training to promote muscle growth. Let's not forget the half glass of wine he has with dinner every day.

Marchand agreed to have his body monitored by researchers from a French university. Eventually, the results were published in the Journal of Applied Physiology.

The results astounded the researchers as Marchand's training proved that regardless of age, it's possible to improve heart and lung health. It also emphasized that most people will respond well to training. Michael Joyner is a physiologist at the Mayo clinic and had this to say.

"Marchand shows that theoretically that there's no upper age limits to training,"

I couldn't agree more.

One of the key elements to Marchand's success and longevity is that he had a structured fitness program geared to his level of ability. In other words, you do what you can. It makes sense to me that seniors should invest in a professional trainer who will set up an individualized training program for them.

When I was watching a video interview of Marchand following his epic ride, I was struck by how mentally sharp he was. Like many plus 100 athletes, he's a living example of how staying fit and embracing a lifestyle of regular exercise improves the quality of life on many levels.

WALDO McBURNEY (October 3, 1902 – July 8, 2009)

Waldo McBurney of Quinter, Kansas was 65 when he began distance running, and was still running into his 90's. He held many records in Masters Track and Field. He attributed his longevity to always staying busy, and eating the vegetables he grew in his garden. At 104, he still had his driver's license.

McBurney's real claim to fame was that at 103 years old, he was recognized as America's oldest worker. He took care of his bee hives every day, that at one time, produced 6000 pounds of honey. It sold out as fast as he could harvest it. Honey was something else that was always on his dining room table during bee season.

Although he was doing more working than running after he turned 100, McBurney still walked to stay fit.

He insisted on staying fit, and really believed the saying, "use it or lose it!

HIDEKICHI MIYAZAKI(THE GOLDEN BOLT)

It's one thing to stay fit in your senior years, but Hidekichi Miyazaki took it to a whole new level when he set a world record in Koyoto, when he blazed through the 100 meter dash in 42.22 seconds.

Although, everyone in attendance was amazed, Miyazaki was disappointed he didn't run faster.

He told AFP in an interview why he was disappointed.

"I'll have to train harder. Training was going splendidly, so I had set myself a target of 35 seconds. I can still go faster."

Miyazaki is also famous to challenging his hero, Usain Bolt to a 100 meter race.

He credits his longevity to exercising daily, and eating in moderation and chewing food properly.

According to the Guinness Book of Records, Miyazaki didn't take up running until he was in his 90's, when all his friends began passing away.

It goes to prove that it's never too late to embrace fitness and improve your quality of life.

PHYLLIS ROWLEY

At 72 years old, Phyllis Rowley, a retired clerk living in Dudley, U.K. decided she was going to take up karate.

It was her way of getting fitter and in the process, she also learned a lot about self-defence. Rowley enjoyed it so much that over the course of six years, she worked her way through the belt ranks.

When she turned 78 years old, she became the oldest female in the United Kingdom to earn the 1st Dan Black Belt. Currently, her goal is to complete her 2nd Dan Belt.

This amazing senior won more than a black belt and fame. Her quality of life is also pretty amazing. Her muscles remain strong as she turns back the clock on sarcopenia; that will take a way muscle mass if seniors don't make the effort to stay physically strong through exercise.

When asked about her journey through the belt ranks as a senior, Rowley had this to say in an interview with Peak Fitness...

"It's the best thing I've ever done and I absolutely love it! I attend three to four classes every week and it's got to the point where it has now become a way of life. I never expected it to go this far. But I feel much safer and have no problems going out at night on my own ... It certainly beats sitting around moping about, or watching TV all day and so I'd encourage everyone my age and older to get active and take up self-defence too."

SISTER MADONNA BUDER

Sister Madonna was born in St. Louis, Missouri in 1930. When she was 23, she became a nun. At the age of 48, she decided to take up running because "Father John told me it would be good for my mind and body."

As I mentioned earlier in this book, running was still pretty new back in 1977 when Sister Madonna prepared to enter her first race. She actually cleared it with her Bishop, and he gave her his blessing and said,

"Sister, I wish some of my priests would do what you're doing."

The 8.2-mile run would become her very first race.

When hearing about the sport of triathlon for the first time, she just knew she had to give it a try. At the age of 52, she competed in her first triathlon in Banbridge, Ireland.

At 75 years old, she earned the title, Iron Nun when she completed 2005 Ironman Hawaii. The world's most famous endurance event includes a 2.4-mile swim, a 112-mile bike, and a full 26.2-mile marathon.

In 1966, she finished the Ironman distance in 14:27:14 and in the process, set a new world record for the 65-69 age category.

I was in Penticton, B.C., Canada videotaping the finish line in 2012 when Sister Madonna Buder set the world record for the oldest person to ever complete the Ironman distance. What an inspiration this remarkable woman is.

She single-handedly opened up about five age-groups for women that never existed until she appeared on the triathlon scene.

Buder raced in the 85-Plus category in an Omaha, Nebraska Olympic Distance Triathlon, and in her career, she completed 45 Ironman races and a total of 350 triathlons.

FAUJA SINGH

Fauja Singh took up distance running at the age of 89. He'd lived in India all his life until his son was killed in a car accident. Singh then moved to England, and that was where his running career started.

He amazed the sporting world by running a marathon (26.2 miles) that same year in six hours and 54 minutes. He was 58 minutes faster than the record for his age group.

I can remember following the Toronto Marathon online the year Singh completed the race at 100 years old. At 104 years old, he was part of the Mumbai Marathon. In 2004, he also replaced David Beckham as the face of Adidas to endorse the brand.

On April 1, 2017, Singh turned 106. Although, he no longer runs, he walks every day. He was asked what his secret to longevity was, and he had this to say.

"I think what has saved me is that I have no ego and no greed. I have never wanted to hoard any money or create a large bank balance. I exercise

everyday and watch what I eat and resist meaningless temptations.

Now a days, people start using a walking stick soon after they turn 60. Look at me - I've never used a walking stick. Yes, with time my vision and hearing have deteriorated, but I'm very fit for my age."

He also said *"I still walk everyday - I know that I will be finished if I stop walking."*

That, in a nutshell, is the essence of this book.

Do your best to keep moving, and challenging your body to stay strong, and you can have the potential to live years longer with an amazing quality of life.

All these stories, and hundreds more just like them about seniors around the world have one thing in common. All these seniors never stopped. They never equated getting older with getting slower. They never gave in to the natural degeneration of their bodies that far too many people accept as just the way it is.

Although, there are no guarantees about how long we'll live, there is always the opportunity to give ourselves the best chance, and improve our quality of life and longevity. Walk, run, swim, bike, or lift those weights.

Find your groove.

Do what you love.

Just never stop moving.

END

OTHER BOOKS BY THE AUTHOR

Ironstruck...The Ironman Triathlon Journey

Ironstruck...500 Ironman Triathlon Questions and Answers

Triathlete In Transition(for beginner triathletes)

Lifestruck...A better way for today's youth

When Running Is Not Enough(Author athletic career biography)

163

Manufactured by Amazon.ca
Bolton, ON

36157220R00090